For

Helen Rechner
and
Kay Karras' sister
a darling author who
writes the most
amazing limericks
in the world.

Helen, herself, is
famous author
who won a new
1955 Ford Sedan

Congratulations!

Fondly,

Dorothy
& Buddie

Editing, Layout and Cover Design: Judith James.

Copy Editing: Leslie Ione Leraan

Cover Photo: Dorothy Hutchinson Welker at age 17 in 1923.

Interior Photos provided by Dorothy Welker - Greengard.

First edition published in 1996

by

Paper Moon Publishing

To order additional copies of Hen Medic,
send $9.95 plus $1.50 S&H *($11.45 total) to:

Paper Moon, Inc.
7230 S. Cnty. Rd. P.,
Lake Nebagamon, WI 54849

***If you reside in Wisconsin,
please add .55¢ tax ($12.00 total).**

Printed in USA on
Elemental Chlorine Free paper
by IMAGE PRESS
14550 28th Avenue North
Minneapolis, MN 55447
800-509-5556

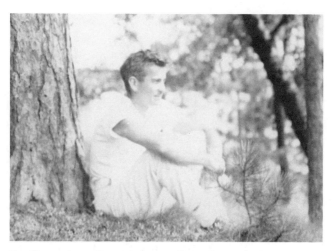

Dedicated to the memory of Dr. Joseph Greengard,
my dear husband.

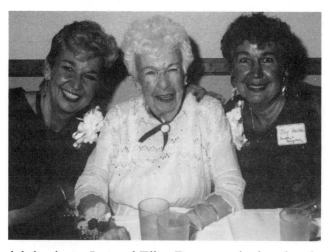

Special thanks to Joy and Ellen Dove, my loving daughters.

~

Also, I am most grateful to Judi James and C.J. Swanson for their
enthusiasm, encouragement and diligence.

HEN MEDIC

Woman Doctor Indeed!

by

Dorothy Hutchinson - Welker, MD

Paper Moon Publishing
Paper Moon, Inc.
Lake Nebagamon, WI

PROLOGUE

"Ladies and gentlemen, your cadavers await you."
I glanced into the room apprehensively. Rows and rows of still figures wrapped in layers of cheesecloth lay on tables on each side of a wide aisle at the far end of which were six narrow, dirt encrusted windows.

Barbara and I shuddered and kept walking toward the far distant window. A strong smell of formaldehyde mixed with the sweetish smell of decay engulfed us, I felt nauseated.

I reached out tentatively to touch the cadaver on the right. I knew I had to feel for good muscles, but I shrank from the task. I looked across at Barbara who smiled encouragingly. She liked my choice.

I reached my hand out once more, grasped the cadaver's arm and nearly fainted. It was WARM! It took me several minutes to realize the arm was room temperature and that my hand was ice cold. Could there be anything worse than this?

The boys came crowding in and I was glad when Kenny found me and approved of my choice. The cadaver looked like a sailor with large tatoo marks on his arms and chest. We named him Barnacle Bill. I wondered what happened to the sailor to have died so young and unemaciated. It was very exciting now that the first shock was over. We pretended that we were pathologists doing an autopsy on a puzzling case.

The little instructor suddenly appeared at our table.

"Do the lower arms and hands first, doctors," he said with sarcasm. "Every muscle must be cleanly dissected so that you can demonstrate the origins and insertions of each one." He noticed the surgical gloves that I was wearing. "Afraid to get your hands dirty? Such a lady! Whoever told you that you could be a doctor?"

I looked straight into his squinty little eyes: "My father, Professor Welker," I told him, matter of factly.

Dr. Weinstein appeared puzzled and then suddenly enlightened and embarrassed. He lowered his head and sidled away crab-like.

"That's telling him!" said Kenny, going back to his dissection. "He's a real creep."

I laughed. I had won my first encounter with woman doctor prejudice. Also, the amused expression in Kenny's kind, hazel eyes helped.

When we were dating in Urbana-Champaign, Kenny had persuaded me to watch an operation, a thyroidectomy by the great thyroid surgeon, Dr. Percy. We climbed up into the high balcony over looking the operating pit.

I had heard about the students fainting at the first operation, so I was very proud of feeling fine as I looked at the gaping wound in the patient's neck. It was almost eight inches across and surrounded by dozens of shining, stainless steel hemostats used to stop the bleeding. I grasped the bar in front of me.

Kenny was engrossed in the technique of the operation, explaining it all to me.

I tried to see over the shoulders of the residents assisting Dr. Percy, but all I could see was the huge red hole in the patient's neck. Thank goodness for general anesthesia, I thought.

Then Dr. Percy's voice rose to question the patient: "How do you feel?"

I thought, The patient is asleep. How can she hear him? But the woman could, because she answered, "Just fine, doctor."

It was too much for me. I felt very warm and my hands and

feet prickled – both tell-tale signs. The next thing I knew, I woke up flat on my back in the men's room with Kenny pouring a glass of water on my face.

"What happened?" I asked weakly.

"You fainted, you chicken you," said Kenny, chuckling gleefully. "Didn't you know the whole operation was done under local?"

I sat up, patted the water from my face and sighed.

"Oh Kenny, I'll never be a doctor!"

~ 1923 ~

It was an early June day. The first fragrance of spring had become the heady scent of summer, mingling the sharpness of nasturtiums with the sweetness of honeysuckle.

I lay on a cot on the second floor verandah and enjoyed the delightful country perfumes blown to me on a faint breeze. Strong, old grape vines climbed up the balcony supports and drooped over the white railing. The new, heart-shaped leaves were shiny and green with tiny, curled tendrils between them, a promise of fruit to come. It was good to be seventeen and looking forward to two months' summer vacation at my grandfather's home in Red Hill, Pennsylvania.

I stretched my arms above my head and looked at my pale hands. I hoped I would have a tan by the end of summer; I had made such plans! On rainy days, I would read many of the hither-to-forbidden books in my father's bedroom. Father had always been a *bookaholic,* collecting many types of literature, and I shared this passion with him.

Father's Ph.D. was in physiological chemistry. This year, before I left to join my mother who had gone to Red Hill ahead of me, my father had given me permission to explore any and all of his library. It made me feel so blissfully grown up. Quite an accomplishment, I thought, for a seventeen year-old girl.

Besides reading, on sunny days I would explore

Grandfather's small farm and then come home to eat Grandmother's delicious, Pennsylvania Dutch meals. I would wear ragged jeans and go barefoot every chance I had, and I'd go fishing. I had wanted to run down to the Perkiomen River as soon as I arrived, but there were the usual obstacles, the rods still at the depot and licenses to be bought. Why did I always have to wait so long for things I wanted? I could almost hear Grandfather saying, "Patience child, patience!"

If there was anything that made me want to scream, it was being told to be patient! I thought of Grandfather standing erect and white-haired outside the Red Hill Station, waiting to pick me up upon my arrival. How was it that whenever I didn't see Grandfather for a time, I always forgot what a stern man he was?

He was only five feet five, or six, and yet gave the appearance of much greater height, unbending, determined and with the brightest blue eyes imaginable. He seemed to be looking deep into my soul and, for a moment, I felt as though I was facing the last judgment.

Oh, Grandfather, I thought. If I should ever fail you . . . I couldn't imagine what tragedy might befall if I ever did let my Grandfather down.

We climbed into the buggy and with a brisk slap of the reins on the backs of the horses, the pair was off at a brisk walk.

The tassel of the dashboard whip waved back and forth in the breeze, as though it were a little flag announcing my arrival. Suddenly, the buggy and Grandfather appeared quaint to me, but only for an instant. Somehow, no matter how I tried, I could not think of Grandfather as humorous or even quaint; stern, sturdy, thrifty, intelligent and rigid, but never quaint!

He half turned toward me. "Your father wrote me that he wants you to study medicine. Is that right?"

"He thinks it would be a good idea." I responded.

"What do you think about it?"

I almost replied, "It doesn't seem to matter," but changed it to, "I hope I'll be able to do it."

"If you are anything like your Father, you will be all right. He made the best showing on his Ph.D. examinations of any candidate at Columbia. I suppose he was sorry he could not complete his MD requirements, too."

"Yes," I agreed, "I guess he couldn't afford that and a wife too." I was going to get my MD no matter what obstacles stood in my way! I wondered whether Grandfather would explain why he had not given the necessary financial backing for my father's MD requirements, but he remained aloof. Perhaps he had been thinking, *enough is enough*. He probably saw no necessity for further study once Father married. That would have been against his native thrift.

I turned over and looked again at the sturdy grapevines climbing over the verandah railing. They were old, dependable and productive like the Welker family. Generations of farmers, teachers and ministers; all sensible, intelligent, Pennsylvania Dutch. It made a fitting background for a doctor. But was I a *typical* Welker?

I hated the words "sensible" and "respectable", heard so often in my father's conversations. I wondered if it were right to pretend to be enthusiastic about my medical education when I really felt rather ambiguous about my immediate future. Leaving home in Oak Park, for undergraduate studies at the University of Illinois in Urbana was a frightening prospect.

Well, one thing sure, I was not going to let my summer be spoiled by all these troublesome doubts. This little break in my studies was going to be enjoyed to the fullest.

I stood up and looked over the hilly countryside. There was Grandmother's garden, with its high banked beds and deep paths and just beyond it spread the plum and apple orchards. Past a patch work of fields at the foot of a wooded hill was a cluster of hardwoods with a brook running through it.

Why worry about the future? After all, there would be a whole summer before I would be a premedic. I ran down the stairs, through the orchard, down, down, down . . . past corn and wheat and clover to my special spot by the brook. Twenty feet away from it, I knelt down and crept forward cautiously.

Would he still be there under the cut bank, my own brown trout? I knew from past encounters that one vibration of the earth would make him disappear so I held my breath, inching forward in slow motion.

I hoped, I believed. Yes, there he was longer, heavier and as smug as ever, facing upstream with his fins and tail waving gently in the current. I was glad that the two of us were alive and there, I on the bank and he in his home, reenacting my childhood happiness. To feel, to breathe, to be free to do what I wanted – this was living.

I spent the afternoon with Grandfather collecting tolls, and enjoying the scenery together, one of the few pleasures we shared. We rode over the red clay roads, up and down the rounded delightful hills. Grandfather gave a short staccato nod whenever we passed a farmer. Most of them called his name aloud and waved with a full arm sweep as they walked behind their plow horses. I wondered how many of them were especially cordial because of the mortgages in Grandfather's possession.

Pennsylvania was striated with byways, crisscrossing counties where extra finances were needed to repair the simple, two lane dirt roads. Some of them were owned by local business men, like my grandfather, and others belonged to the county. In both cases the gates were tended by toll keepers who lived in small frame houses next to them. When a vehicle drew near, the toll keeper, or his wife would appear to collect the money and open the gate. Then, once a month, the tolls were turned in to the owners.

At our first toll station, a thin dark haired man thrust his head out of a second-story window and pulled it in just as quickly. Three dirty, barefoot little girls stepped shyly around the corner of the house and stood in a questioning row. Their forefingers were in their mouths, the hems of their dresses uneven.

I smiled at them, but they stared back with an apathy through which kindness was not felt. The front door was flung open. The toll keeper ran out and hurriedly deposited a clinking small cloth bag in Grandfather's outstretched hand.

"Veir und fünfstick."

Four and fifty, the amount he stated, was my concern. I counted it then noted it in what I hoped was the right column.

"Grosdanke," Grandfather's thank you, and we were off.

"Why are toll keepers always so dirty?" I asked.

Grandfather did not answer until I repeated the question.

"Because they are poor — and the poor are dirty," he answered callously.

"Can't the county pay them more?" I asked, knowing I was tempting his anger.

"They get a house to live in and a patch to grow vegetables and raise chickens on. What more can they want? It's better than the poorhouses where we get them from, isn't it?"

I noticed he was chewing on the edge of his small white mustache and, since I knew this to mean retreat was called for, I meekly agreed.

"Take the cigar worker," he continued, "They are always trying to get more money, but the owners cannot make any profit that way. If we stick together and keep all wages within reason, these people will stop getting fancy ideas."

I wondered what fancy ideas those three little girls could possibly have had.

We rode in silence until we came to a ford. The wagon tracks went perpendicular into the clay bottom creek. Charlie, the graying chestnut gelding, splashed in happily and stopped in midstream. He lowered his head to take in great, snorting gulps of the cold water. Grandfather let the reins hang loose while he looked up and down stream.

"The fish are rising pretty well," he said. "I suppose I'll have to take you and your Grandmother fishing."

I was happy for there was nothing I liked better than fishing in the Perkiomen River. My father was the expert fisherman in the family and organized many expeditions, but when he was away, as he was now, a fishing trip was a rare and unexpected pleasure.

I was glad when Grandfather picked up the reins and gave Charlie an admonishing slap. I could hardly keep from laughing.

"When Grandaudy, please, when?"

He smiled quietly at hearing my pet name for him. "Well, we'll see."

I had to be content with that – darn it.

On Monday, Grandfather was too busy collecting the weekend tolls and sorting the mail and still made no mention of fishing, so I spent the day working in the store.

Built long before the Civil War, my grandparent's home was large and well constructed of heavy, gray stone native to the area. Wood trim painted sparkling white, surrounded the windows and doors. One third of the structure was a general store and post office with a delivery platform on the side and offices on the second floor.

I enjoyed working in the store, although many of the customers spoke only Pennsylvania Dutch so I had difficulty talking with them. Often I had to call my aunt or mother into the store to translate for me.

Large, built-in, wooden bins held flour, dried fruit, coffee beans, tea, sugar and other dry goods. The best was the dark brown sugar with delicious lumps which I filched and ate when no one was watching. That is until one of my cousins caught me and teased, saying, "The lumps are made by the farm hands spitting on it."

I didn't believe my cousin's story, but somehow I could never nibble those lumps again.

There were bolts of gingham and calico and fascinating glass-doored cabinets with drawers of thread in colors to match the dress goods. There were yards and yards of braid and ribbons and bindings that made me itch to sew. Naturally Grandfather stocked needles and pins and pretty little silver and gold thimbles, sparkling like tiny treasures.

There were gleaming rows of clear glass jars with round glass tops like sparkling crowns above their contents of pink and white striped mints, colorful jelly beans and shining, black licorice strips so fresh and chewy that each lasted ten minutes.

My favorite job in the store was weighing out bulk items on the sturdy scale for that purpose. I was always careful to place a piece of white wrapping paper in the wire basket on the left hand side of the scale − to keep clean whatever I was weighing. Next I would choose from the perfectly contoured series of ten, five, one pound and little one ounce brass weights, placing the correct amount on the right side of the scale. Then, came the truly fun part − scooping the dry goods into the basket until the scale balanced.

The large, red coffee mill was fun to turn and, because the customers preferred freshly ground coffee, there was a lot of grinding to be done. This apparatus made a terrific racket, but the rich, strong aroma of coffee it gave off was heavenly.

There were large wooden barrels filled with spicy things like huge, garlic pickles, salty herring and, best of all, sauerkraut made fresh every week. These items had to be weighed, too, and that wasn't as much fun. I hated having to weigh a smoked perch or mackerel, so shiny, stiff and *smelly*.

Most people charged their purchases and I had to write each item, its cost and the total on the individual's own page in a long gray account book, smudged with many penciled entries. On payday, the cigar workers from the nearby factory lined up to make a payment on their bills, but some of them had stopped on the way to have a few drinks at the saloon and so could not pay all they owed.

When Grandfather was in the store, they sidled up sheepishly and handed him a few large dollar bills which he took with a tart remark, "Next time, it would be better to come directly here without any side trips."

I couldn't understand why they never seemed to resent this mild scolding. I thought perhaps they did, but did not dare show it, as Grandfather probably would have discontinued their charge accounts. Yes, I was sure that would be just the sort of thing Grandfather would do.

Later during that first day back at work in Grandfather's store, there was a lull in business and I wondered why customers usually came in bunches. It would have been so much more convenient if they came in one at a time, instead of arriving in groups of four or five, almost filling the small space between the counters.

When the store emptied out, I climbed up the three steps behind the counter near the entrance to where the roll top desk commanded a good view of the entire store. That was where the locked cash box was kept in a very secret drawer opened only by pressing on a spring in a side panel.

It always made me sad to sit at this desk because it reminded me of Aunt Annie, a friendly and charming woman with a warm smile and the softest lap imaginable. She died when I was six, but left an indelible memory of happy hours spent sitting with her at this old oak desk while she drew funny stick animals with large grins on their faces.

I went through the side door of the store into the long, low dining room of the house proper. To the right, was the new kitchen which Grandfather had supplied with the most up to date equipment: a gas stove with two ovens, long wooden counters just the right height for kneading bread, and a shining white ice chest which opened from the top to show a place for a large cake of ice with room around the sides for milk, cream and butter from our three Guernsey cows.

The rest of the family's food was kept in the cold cellar, a damp dark hole in the ground. I ventured down the twelve frighteningly steep steps leading down to rows and rows of open cabinets. It seemed to me that the shelves were always filled with glass jars of Grandmother's homemade *everything* – including sauerkraut, pickled beets and creamed corn.

How my grandmother found time to plant, grow, cook and can all this produce was beyond my imagination. There were also bins of potatoes, carrots and apples among other things. And there was that one special kind of apple that was a little bigger than a crab and a little smaller than a winesap, that brought me down to the spooky cold cellar. They grew abundantly in Grandmother's orchard, but I never was able to find the variety anywhere else. It was tart, crisp and yummy!

I climbed back outdoors through the heavy trap door while happily munching my unknown apple. The garden smelled mysteriously sweet and delightful, as usual. I could never identify the separate odors, but altogether they made an almost overwhelming, wonderful scent. I spent the rest of the day becoming reacquainted with the sights, sounds and smells I loved. Everywhere I turned, I was reminded of the people most dear to me.

Grandmother's garden was a sight to behold. She spent all her mornings among her flowers and vegetables. In return for this meticulous, nurturing care they bloomed and produced like no other garden in the neighborhood.

Over the years, she put so much fertilizer and good black dirt on the beds that the paths between them were over a foot deep. It made the weeding and picking at a convenient height for the little old lady. It was difficult for me to think of Grandmother as old, however. She was so active and quick and erect that she never seemed her age.

She could do more in a day than anyone else I knew. According to people who could understand Pennsylvania Dutch, she never grumbled about her work or criticized anyone. She had a pixie smile, with the corners of her eyes wrinkled up and the edges of her lips tucked in like those of a little chipmunk. Her happiest hours were spent fishing. That's probably what I liked most about her. She was awaiting the promised fishing trip as eagerly as I.

When the day arrived, I couldn't eat much breakfast in anticipation of the event of which I had dreamed of all through the snowy, Oak Park winter. I cleared the dishes from the table and helped make sandwiches and hot black coffee for the picnic lunch. Grandfather was calling from the back door.

"Hurry up you women. Aren't you ready yet?"

Fishing was an unnecessary waste of time for him, but he tolerated it once in awhile because *Der Kin* seemed to enjoy it so much. Usually I resented being called a child, but did not mind anything at a time like this.

"We're coming, Grandaudy," I answered.

We climbed into the buggy loaded with a checkered tablecloth, napkins, large jugs of lemonade and coffee, picnic baskets, fishing poles and cans of earthworms. Mother stayed behind to mind the store.

It was a seemingly endless, half-hour drive to the Perkiomen River. The covered, wooden bridge that meant we were finally there was a welcome sight when it appeared around the bend of the road.

The Perkoimen River, a peaceful, moderate-sized stream meandered quietly between high cut banks where small mouth bass lay. The liquid gurgling over rocks and fallen tree trunks mingled with the sharp banter of red winged black birds calling to each other. The delicious smells of the new mown hay in the field made me want to roll in it.

Aunt Alice, who never fished, being too dainty to soil her delicate hands with bait, was placed on a blanket under a huge walnut tree. She was delegated to call us at noon for lunch. In the meantime, she contentedly read her church pamphlets and arranged her long skirt modestly over her ankles. I often thought Aunt Alice had been born a spinster.

Grandmother and I wasted no time finding our favorite place on the embankment of the south side of the bridge where the water carried our lines downstream. We loaded our medium-sized hooks with juicy red earthworms, above which we placed large lead sinkers, three feet from the medium size corks.

Side by side, we settled down, breathlessly watching our bobbing corks. Grandmother taught my father to fish and now she was teaching me the skills needed to perfect my already instilled desire. I loved to see her pull up the long bamboo pole with all her might whenever her cork went under, often losing her sunbonnet in the excitement, and it wasn't long before I saw just such a scene.

We rejoiced over her catch and Grandmother's cheeks glowed with the pleasure of her accomplishment. It seemed we didn't even need words to share our delight. We placed the small-mouth bass on a stringer hung from the bridge and went back to catching more.

We hated to stop fishing when Aunt Alice ordered us to come and eat. We compromised by propping our poles against the bridge railing and weighing them down with large rocks so that no monstrous carp could make off with the tackle. We watched the tips of the bamboo poles and, if one dipped down suddenly, we made a mad dash to rescue it and capture the prize dangling at the end of the line, glittering in the noonday sun.

Aunt Alice shook her head in disgust at such "carryings on," but Grandmother and I just laughed.

Many such idyllic days, surrounded by those I loved most in the world, filled my summer sojourn. Even so, it seemed over much too soon when my last Sunday in Grandfather's house dawned with a pearly gray light creeping into my bedroom.

I dressed with reluctance, thinking the discomfort of leaving my warm bed was a large price to pay for the doubtful satisfaction of attending church services. I shivered as I dressed; my clothes were slightly damp from the dew that seeped through the open windows during the night. I brushed my hair vigorously in an effort to awaken my sleep-dulled senses. I was never ready to go to bed at night and hated to get up in the morning.

I gave a last, defiant brush stroke. What a time to start for church, six-thirty! Those who went willingly at that hour surely must be patient, docile persons in need of no further saving. For a rebellious soul such as I, the insult of that untimely arising made me even more resistant to salvation.

As I entered the long, low dining room, the aroma of simmering chicken enveloped me. Preparations for the midday meal were being made in the old kitchen, for this meal had to be ready before everyone left for church.

The old kitchen was a dark little hole filled with a large, dingy table and chairs. The pine paneling was smoke-stained from many years of previous meals. Above the lower half of the paneled walls, separated by a chair-rail, hung old-fashioned, blue and white checked wall paper.

The family breakfast was solemn, with Grandfather murmuring, "Be present at out table, Lord, be here and everywhere adored. Thy creatures bless and grant that we may feast in paradise with Thee."

I half opened my eyes while he prayed and looked at Grandmother with great admiration. This lady of seventy, still young in appearance, was made up of a series of curves – a small round head, two half-spheres for breasts, plump little hands clasped over a most dignified, round abdomen. Even her feet were small and plump. She was wearing a blue and white dress with a starched white apron pulled in tight around her waist.

Grandmother and I could not converse well because I spoke very little Pennsylvania Dutch and she did not know English. However, in spite of this language barrier, we were most companionable. We spent many hours in peaceful silence, with only a gesture or a smile to compliment one another on a task well done.

When breakfast was over, Grandmother disappeared to change quickly and expertly into her Sunday best – stiff, black, rustling taffeta with narrow black lace edging the high neck and cuffs. Her small, black, poke bonnet was tied under her chin and was trimmed with two purple velvet pansies, a daring innovation. She sat quietly on her own horsehair rocking chair in the corner, while my aunt, my mother and I gathered our going-to-church possessions.

Grandfather, splendid in a black alpaca suit, starched white shirt and neatly-tied, black, string bow tie, stood in the doorway snapping and unsnapping his heavy-chained, gold pocket watch. It was a signal to the women folk to stop fussing around and get ready to leave immediately.

"Die Mom," he said, "Dut sich of und schtelt sich auf die ecke" which pointedly reminded us of Grandmother's good example for it told us, "The Mother dresses herself and stands herself in the corner."

Despite my earlier reluctance, I enjoyed the long and lovely trip to church. The family-filled buggy, pulled by two bay horses, traveled briskly over narrow, winding, red, clay roads. Farm lay next to farm, with well kept fences marking their boundaries. The rounded, patchwork hills in shades of green stretched away to the horizon where greater hills appeared bluish-violet and mysterious.

Particularly, I liked the large red barns with the "hex" over their hayloft doors. These symmetrically painted designs were supposed to keep all bad luck away. The huge barns appeared sturdy and overwhelming beside the meek, insignificant, white farmhouses. Those formidable barns and the smaller buildings of the homesteads reminded me that here, in this particular section of Southeastern Pennsylvania during the first quarter of the twentieth century, Father ruled the family, or at least he thought he did.

The Old Goschenhoppen Dutch Reformed Church had been built in pre-Revolutionary days. It had three-foot-thick gray, native stone walls just like Grandfather's house. It graced a high hill with simplicity and grandeur. We approached it on foot, having tied the horses in the open white sheds that were partially hidden by a clump of maple trees at the foot of the hill.

As we climbed the painfully steep slope, I thought that the first minister must have planned the approach this way, because as we stopped for breath we could look at the surrounding tombstones and meditate on death. Thus, we entered the church in a properly chastened mood.

That particular minister had always been a special object of hero worship during my childhood because of the story told to me about the time he said, "In seventeen hundred and seventy-five, there is a time to pray and a time to fight." Whereupon, he threw open his vestments and revealed an American Revolutionary uniform underneath. I liked to think of him stepping down from the pulpit and striding grandly off to the war.

We four women sat quietly in the Welker pew to the left of the aisle. The men and boys of the congregation sat on benches lined up lengthwise to the main aisle on the right side of the church. Men and women were never allowed to sit side by side in God's house.

The inside of the church was coldly chaste with one simple painting on the wall behind the pulpit depicting Christ ascending into heaven on a feather-beddish cloud.

The services that Sunday were in German so the effect on my rebellious spirit was worse than if I had attended the alternate English Sunday. My time was spent looking out the window and observing the love life of several amorous dragonflies

The long moments passed slowly by with the unknown expostulation of the minister, reiterating like a drawn out chant to my uncomprehending ears. This priceless Sunday was being wasted listening to a drone. Up and down, inflection followed inflection. Although at first I rebelled against these meaningless sounds, I began to feel an overpowering, emotional sensation descend on me like a cloak upon unwilling shoulders. I was enveloped in peace. I looked about and saw almost everyone settled back into a satisfied half-coma.

The sun shone through the open eastern window and a large horsefly buzzed persistently against the upper pane. It provided a distraction to save me from the persistent drone. I didn't realize then what hypnotic effect a voice could have. Only later, when I would be exposed to the practice of hypnotism, would I wonder if half of this congregation weren't under a hypnotic spell every Sunday.

There was a quick rustling among the worshippers as they emerged from their pleasant stupor and reached for the hymnals in the racks on the back of the pews ahead of them. The closing hymn at last! I stood up and as I held one side of Mother's hymnal. I tried to pronounce the German words. I noticed that Mother, as usual, was not singing in church. Whenever I asked her why, she always replied, "Because I do not sing well enough." Yet, she had a pleasant tuneful voice whenever she sang at home.

Suddenly, as I stood beside my silent mother, I wondered whether her refusal to sing was a manifestation of some inner revolt against religion. My peaceful mood was disturbed by something aloof and unreceptive about my mother that was entirely alien to her nature. "Mother?" I whispered, as if tentatively trying to draw out a vague figure which I could not quite discern in the shadow.

Mother turned her head towards me and her expression softened to one of enfolding tenderness.

"Yes?" she answered.

"Oh, nothing." I was reassured by the familiar expression of love and warmth. Tomorrow I would leave Grandfather's house. I was facing enough uncertainty without questioning my mother's character.

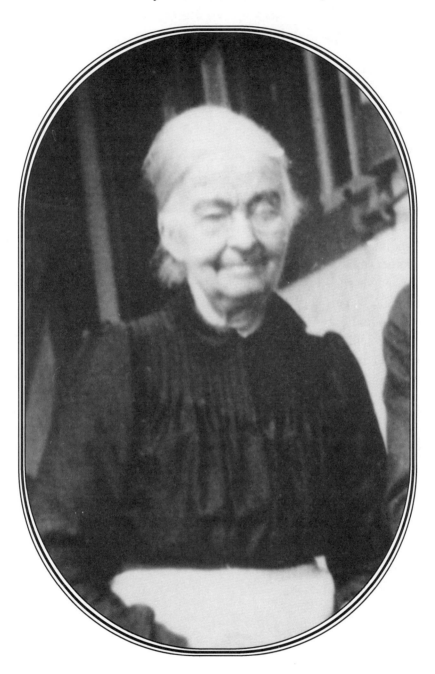

Grandmother Welker

DOWNSTATE

I said good-bye to my grandparents and my mother, who was staying on a while longer, as Father was still so occupied with his research on rattlesnake venom, and took the train back home to Oak Park. Now, Father was taking me to what would turn out to be the first leg of my life's journey.

The ponderous, family automobile moved majestically down the Chicago boulevards. The car, the buildings, everything was such a contrast to the simplicity of Red Hill. My pleasant respite in Red Hill had ended too soon.

I held my purse and gloves in cold hands. Father was driving to the Northwestern Railroad Station for my first trip away from home alone. He seemed oblivious to my trepidation. There he sat with his hat on correctly straight and his top coat buttoned up to the neck. I touched his arm, but he did not look at me as I had hoped. Instead, he half-growled, "What's the matter? Buck fever?"

"I suppose so." I answered in resignation to his stoic nature.

We drove a few more miles. I glanced at my wristwatch. I wished we would be late for the train so I could postpone my departure until the next morning. Leaving in late afternoon was a miserable time. I had not been able to eat any lunch nor did I sleep well the two previous nights.

I hated my father's determination for me to be a doctor. I

was an only child and a poor substitute for the boy he had always wanted. Still, Father was always kind to. He wouldn't insist I go away to school if I objected in any way. Right then, I wished I had protested, but the truth was I'd never dreamed of opposing my father.

As Father drove me closer to my fate, I wished I could tell him − blurt out my fears, but we only sat side by side, silent in our thoughts, each doing what we thought best for the other. If this was the way all great adventures started, I wanted no part of them! I trembled as I looked about and saw we were entering the gloomy environs of the station.

My father parked the car, backing in with the same precise skill with which he did everything. It was maddening! If only he would commit one rash act, lose his temper, throw something at someone or break a window, I would feel closer to him in moments like these. He was too perfect in my estimation and I felt so unperfected.

He glanced at me, his eyes scrutinizing, then registering kindly concern. "Feel all right?"

I felt like a wretch for the things I had been thinking. I had to say something. I knew he was expecting me to.

He repeated, "Dorothy, are you feeling ill?"

I knew he wanted me to be brave. "I'm fine. I'll be all right when I get on the train."

He reached into his inside coat pocket and handed me the things I'd need for my journey − a gesture that recalled my youth. I felt like a dependent child no more than ten years old.

"Tickets, checkbook, money, directions for registration. I'm sure you'll find them all in order."

I knew I would when my father gave them to me. I pushed them into my purse and ran after him. He was already carrying my bags down the street. I wanted to cry out, to call him back, in some way stop the progression of this day. Panic swept over me as the remorseless inevitability of going away penetrated my consciousness.

I was sure Father had never had a moment like this, so how could he possibly understand? I ran stumbling after him feeling lost and alone.

Inside, the station was crowded, horribly filled with coal smoke and soot and laughing people. They all seemed very happy, pleased with their private circumstances. Their mirth was such a contrast to my utter despair.

Father and I began climbing the steep stairs to the upper level where the trains were made up. A wave of nausea engulfed me. I tried ignoring it but, could not.

"Father," I said.

He turned and really looked at me. He saw that I was pale.

"Here now, Dorothy," he said. "A coed can't faint; that's mid-Victorian."

I wanted to smile at his deliberate use of my favorite term of disdain, but I just couldn't.

He piloted me firmly to a door marked LADIES.

"If there ever wasn't a lady, that's me!" I thought. I disappeared inside and succumbed to my nausea, retching what little was in my stomach. When I'd regained my composure, I returned to Father and we went to the train without further delay.

The rail car was as crowded as the station, jammed with exuberant youths. None of them ever seemed to be stationary; running in the aisles, slapping each other on the back, starting card games, throwing luggage on the racks. It was one seething mass of constant motion.

I felt more alone than ever, now that Father had gone. I huddled into as small a space as possible and stared out of the train window, facing the bleak, soot-smeared, station wall opposite me. One bright light bulb shone back, hurting my eyes. The nausea had passed and in its place was a vast ache. If I were homesick now, even before I left Chicago, what would school be like?

The train started with a lunge, causing wild glee among the other passengers. I only felt like crying. A loud cheer exploded and then they began singing something that ended with "Chicago for her Standard Oil, for good fellows, Illinois."

The click of the wheels on the rails, the sideways sway of the cars and the singing seemed to have a calming effect and I relaxed a bit for the first time in three days. The conductor passing by reached over and gently extracted the ticket I held in my half-opened hand. I sighed and settled back, placing my cheek against the window sill.

The ride along the bumpy rails took about three hours, so I was happy when the courteous conductor gently awoke me by touching my shoulders and I realized I'd slept through most of it.

"Wake up little lady," he said. "Welcome to Urbana - Champaign, the home of the University of Illinois downstate."

I thanked him and gathered my purse, hatbox, suitcase and laundry box and made my way off the train. I found a porter who carried my things the rest of the way to a waiting taxi-cab. The ride to the university campus was uneventful. Once there, I followed behind the taxi driver who was laden with my belongings.

We arrived at the ladies' dorm. Tall white columns against a red brick facade, four stories and quite substantial, it starkly contrasted with our small, tan frame house in Oak Park. As if to further accentuate the difference from anything familiar, the heavy colonial door opened and a little old woman stood there looking at me. I assumed her to be the housemother, but she was as unlike my mother as she could possibly be.

Her puckered face was smiling with every wrinkle. She held out her hand. I took it tentatively.

"I am Daisy Blaisdell, my dear, your housemother," the woman said in a very New England voice. "Welcome to Urbana."

"Thank you," I said and stepped inside. Miss Blaisdell put an arm around my shoulders and I discovered the unexpectedly reassuring fact that my housemother was no taller than myself.

"I'm Dorothy Welker," I answered the unspoken question.

"From?"

"From Oak Park."

"Oh yes, a very lovely suburb." My home was approved, at any rate. "Your father is Professor Welker from the professional school?"

"Yes," I answered. She was referring to the Medical, Dental and Pharmacy Departments of the Chicago Campus. "I suppose Dean Myer, from the graduate school, told you."

Miss Blaisdell smiled coyly, "Oh, I have all sorts of advance information about my girls. Let me take you up to your room."

She led the way up the wide carpeted stairs between handsome, white painted and polished mahogany banisters.

"You are indeed fortunate to have such a charming young lady for a roommate, Edna Darcy from Rockford," she said, opening the door to what would be my room for the next few months.

I looked around my new home. It was a corner room, large and light, with six windows and a wide window seat under three of them. Two cots, two mirrored closets, two desks and several comfortable chairs suggested all sorts of decorative possibilities. A suitcase on one of the cots told me my roommate had been there and gone.

"Edna is attending a rushing tea this afternoon," Miss Blaisdell smiled in a satisfied way, as though it were a triumph of her own. "Well, I'll leave you now, my dear - er, Dorothy," she said with an obvious effort to remember my name. "Please come down for dinner at the second chime." She started out of the room with a quick, bird-like motion, her head tilted to one side and a shiny eye still examining me, even as she sidled through the door.

I didn't know whether or not I liked my new housemother and decided that the feeling probably was mutual.

I examined the room more closely. Apparently, Edna had lost no time in claiming her turf, because she had placed her suitcase on the cot situated out of the draft, her belongings in both top dresser drawers and her clothes in the most convenient closet.

I sighed and sat down on the remaining cot, too discouraged to move. This was a far cry from the home in which I was an only child with everything revolving about me. After a few minutes, I shrugged off my self pity and started unpacking, but I'd be darned if I would give up everything without a struggle.

I carefully removed Miss Edna Darcy's belongings from one of the top dresser drawers and deposited them firmly and finally in a bottom drawer. "There," I said to myself, "If this is to be a boxing match, I'll make it a good one!"

The cot and closet I conceded as round one and two, claiming the dresser as a draw in round three. "But there will be more rounds, be'gorry."

The first chime sounded. I found the bathroom at the end of the hall and washed my hands and face. Several pleasant, excited young girls were tidying up for dinner. I liked their friendly greetings and felt more at home. One pretty, blonde girl with braids around her head was called "Frenchy," because she looked like a French doll. She had a pink and white complexion with a tiny little nose. I would find out that her innocent, blue-eyed stare hid a devilish imagination and a daring spirit that refused to turn down any challenge. She would become the ringleader of our gang of six; Nita, June, Ike, Emote, Frenchy and myself. A group with marvelous rapport, we would be dubbed, *The Sinful Six.*

I went down to dinner alone, because I was a little slower than the rest of the girls, having to wait until they were finished. The second chime sounded while I was still washing up.

The dining room was in the basement, a dark unattractive room with many long tables. At the end of the head table sat Miss Blaisdell, regally dignified and bestowing her conversation on favorites who sat beside her. Her assistant, Miss Carson, as I was told by the girl seated at my right, was stationed at the head of another long table. She was a peasant-like woman, with a motherly expression and a large bosom. I judged her to be in her late forties. I liked her looks.

The meal was starchy with macaroni and cheese as the entree. For beverage, we had our choice of lemonade or mild tea. Dessert was a particularly insipid pineapple tapioca. As I took the first mouthful, something gritted between my teeth. I spit it out into my napkin and was horrified to see several pieces of broken glass on top of the pudding. It was just too much.

I dropped my napkin and stumbled up to my room. Suddenly, the whole traumatic day overwhelmed me; leaving home, the train trip, meeting Miss Blaisdell, the unpleasant arrangements of the room, and finally the broken glass in my dessert. I flung myself on my cot and cried. I wished I was home!

In the midst of this turmoil, Edna Darcy appeared, followed by a coterie of three girls. Edna was plump, with a bland, round face and widely-spaced, cool, brown eyes. She looked quite complacent.

"Well," she said, in greeting, "You don't look too happy. Don't you like it here?"

I hated to be put on the defensive. I heartily disliked Edna. Her three tall followers looked decidedly unfriendly.

"Oh," I said, "It will take a bit of getting used to, I guess."

Edna turned to her friends and gave a detailed description of the rushing tea she had just attended. From then on, it was just as though I did not exist.

Later I found my registration schedule and decided to take several required premedic courses, plus an advanced English Literature course. I was allowed to skip English Lit I because of credit from Oak Park and River Forest Township High School. I was glad I had attended this highly accredited school. It permitted all students to skip Freshman English no matter what college or university they attended. I intended to take as many English electives in writing as possible, because I had always enjoyed composing short stories and poetry.

I had been an editor of my school paper and magazine, and a reporter for Oak Leaves, the town newspaper. Of all things, I covered the high school social life. I had always thought that a side benefit of being a doctor was that I could see people with their masks off. This would enable me to understand the characters I wrote about – besides being able to help my patients.

That evening, the first of the weekly house meetings was held. Each girl introduced herself and told where she came from.

I felt particularly attracted to Nita, a small, chic, seventeen year-old with a boyish bob and a piquant turned up nose. She said she came from Matoon, but looked much too cosmopolitan to have come from that small town in Southern Illinois. She walked over to me after the meeting and invited me to a *bull session* in her room after ten p.m., a forbidden time after *lights out.*

It was a delightful few hours, especially appreciated after the chilling reception I had received from my roommate. I shared the details of that ordeal with Nita and the other girls and they expressed immediate sympathy. We all agreed that Edna was a *pill* and they vowed to support me in my battle for space in my room.

The girls were different types: Frenchy was like a little doll, June was dark, tall and spinsterish. Emote was under five feet with big eyes and a wide smile. Her given name was Emily, but the girls nicknamed her Emote because she reacted so emotionally to stimuli. She was a lot of fun. *Ike* was really Irene, the athletic one of the six, with broad shoulders, light brown hair and blue eyes. She had a placid nature, was dependable and pleasant to be with.

These girls were my best friends throughout my years downstate. At times, they were confidants – a shoulder to cry on and at times they were partners in crime. It seems the latter was more often true.

Several months after that first day, I invited two of my male high school friends from Oak Park to come to Urbana for the homecoming prom. Nita agreed to go with one of them to the dance and the two boys convinced us to drive back to Chicago with them the next day. This turned out to be a mistake which I began to worry about as we neared Oak Park.

Father looked amazed as we arrived.

"What are you doing here?" he demanded.

"We thought it would be fun to drive home with the boys. We can catch the train back in the morning." I stammered.

"And what about your Monday classes?"

I swallowed the lump in my throat. "We thought we could cut them."

"Cut classes?" he asked. That was unheard of in the Welker academic philosophy. "You turn right around, drive to the station and catch the next train back today. No arguments!"

Nita clutched at me for support. I felt her arm shaking from fear. The boys were laughing, but to Nita, who had never been threatened in such a menacing tone, this was no laughing matter.

Professor Welker, Chairman of the Admissions and Discipline Committee of the Professional Schools for the University of Illinios was a formidable adversary. He put the fear of God in most of his medical, dental and pharmaceutical students. Single handedly, he could cut-off their professional careers because of any misconduct.

I knew if I was going to be admitted to the University of Illinois College of Medicine, I had to have an exemplary record downstate. I suddenly realized the import of my mistake. I exchanged an understanding glance with my sympathetic mother. Nita and I left immediately, the boys driving us to the railroad station.

Back at Urbana, I had a heavy schedule to contend with — twenty units instead of the customary sixteen, because of my second major in English. My English Literature course required many hours of reading and writing and my long laboratory sessions in my science courses were quite tiring. It was especially difficult because I couldn't study in my room with Edna and her friends draped all over the furniture, chatting away and ignoring all pleas from me to, "be a little quieter." They all made fun of me, calling me a "a greasy grind." The bedlam usually continued all day and in the evening until lights out.

Finally, I could stand it no longer. I applied for a single room and, fortunately, was able to get one because the former occupant had dropped out, but the *gang* was incensed at my treatment. So one night, as we were happily munching toast and drinking Cokes, Frenchy suggested a way to pay Edna back for her misdeeds.

"Let's all come back from semester break early, before Edna does, and move all of her things out onto the landing in front of her room," she said.

Frenchy's idea was greeted with howls of delight and without thinking of the possible consequences, we all agreed to do it. We had a great time planning the whole thing. It was to take place at midnight on the eve of the second semester.

Finally, the night came. We tiptoed around, being careful not to slam closets or dresser drawers. Slowly a whole pile of shoes, hats, underwear, dresses and books arose on the landing and topped it with a huge sign: WELCOME HOME EDNA DEAR!

Next dinner time, a grim faced Miss Blaisdell remained standing after the opening grace.

"I am very disappointed in the actions of some of my girls. An event such as this has never happened in the whole history of the Women's Residence Hall. I demand that anyone who knows anything about this terrible act report to me immediately."

She sat down. There was whispering and sly glancing around to see who acted guilty. The Sinful Six had innocent faces, but I felt a hot flush arising at my neckline and extending to the roots of my hair. Whenever I was in any kind of trouble, my darn blushing gave me away.

As I left the dining room, Miss Blaisdell bustled up to me. "Please follow me to my sitting room," she said.

I looked around for my cohorts, but they had all abandoned me!

Miss Blaisdell motioned for me to sit down. I obeyed, taking a chair across the desk from her in her.

"Dorothy, what do you know about this?"

I didn't know what to say. If I admitted it, I would be disciplined; and if I lied, and was caught in the lie, I would be sent to the Dean of Women's office and possibly expelled.

A vision of my father's disappointed face flashed before me. I knew what I must do.

"I did it," I admitted.

Miss Blaisdel seemed well pleased in having been right in her assumption of my guilt. "Why did you do such a thing?" she asked me.

"My life has been miserable this last semester because of Edna and her friends. I never had a moment's peace or happiness since I moved in. I've had to do my studying in the library or the other girls' rooms because Edna's radio was blaring day and night. I asked her many times if she couldn't be a little quieter, but she refused. I decided to get even."

"Not a very lofty motive, especially since the problem was already solved – now that you have your own room. Who helped you?"

I shook my head and remained silent.

Miss Blaisdel hated to be crossed in any way. "If you don't tell me," she said with great seriousness, "I'll take your privileges away from you."

Thinking of the dates I would have to cancel, all the social events I would miss, I remained silent. It was worth it.

After a few moments, Miss Blaisdell remarked, "Go to your room and remain there until you hear from me."

I climbed the stairs slowly, noting that the debris was gone from the top of the landing – probably cleared away by Edna and the three *Green Giants*, as the girls called Edna's friends. Oh well, I was not sorry no matter what. I went into my solitary room and studied in beautiful silence.

Miss Blaisdale withheld my privileges for two months.

The rest of that first year went by in a hurry with the worry of exams and the fun of dates. There were lots of jokes about the old cemetery where couples went to *neck* because the dating alcoves in the Women's Residence Hall were too closely supervised for even one kiss.

Miss Blaisdell made frequent rounds every evening. Once she came across a boy sprawled on a sofa, talking to his date. She stood in front of him with her arms folded across her chest. "Young man," she said, "Are you ill?"

He rose sheepishly, answering, "Oh, no Ma'am."

"Well," she said decisively, "I thought you must be because I have never seen anyone in that position unless he were ill."

The incident spread throughout the Hall and, by the next day, many girls were saying to each other, "Young woman, are you ill?" and then laughing hilariously.

It was the next fall, when I registered for an elective in psychology, that the Sinful Six nearly found themselves in hot water again.

The psychology instructor, who was particularly interested in hypnosis, gave a demonstration of the technique for his students. It went off well and the boy awoke promptly when the instructor clapped his hands.

I was intrigued with the possibilities of treating patients by means of hypnosis. I imagined myself getting teenagers to stop smoking through the use of post-hypnotic suggestion. So at the next bull session, I described the events of the psychology class to the Sinful Six.

The girls were fascinated by the concept and Emote begged to be hypnotized. I refused.

"Oh please, Dottie!" Emote pleaded, "I've always wondered

what it would be like. Please?"

"I don't know anything about hypnotizing anyone. What if you don't go under?"

"I'll try. I'll try so hard. Please!"

All the girls joined Emote in her efforts to persuade me and, finally, I reluctantly agreed. They formed a circle around the two of us.

I put out all the lights except one candle and talked to Emote in a quiet voice.

"Look at the candle, Emote. I will move it slowly back and forth. As you watch it, you will become drowsy, then drowsier and drowsier. You will relax completely and will slowly fall asleep. You are going to sleep. You are going to sleep. You are going to sleep."

Emote was so anxious to be hypnotized that she fell into a trance-like state in just a few minutes. I lifted up one of her hands and let it go. It dropped back limply onto her lap. I continued. "Close your eyes. You are feeling delightfully relaxed. You are floating on a fluffy cloud. Spread your wings and gently wave them as though flying, but don't leave your chair. You are a bird."

Emote followed my instructions to the letter. The girls stifled amazed giggles. I was delighted with my success.

"Now drop your wings to your sides and walk over to the bed. Make a little nest with the comforter and sit on it." Emote obeyed all commands automatically.

"Now lie down."

Emote settled herself comfortably on the bed, apparently asleep.

I waited about five minutes, time quickly taken up by conversation and comments from the others, and then said, "When I clap my hands three times, you will wake up. You will not remember anything, but you will feel better than you ever have in your life."

I left her alone for another five minutes, distracted by Nita and Frenchy asking for their turns. June and Ike would have no part in it.

"Shall we wake her now?" I asked.

They agreed.

I clapped my hands three times. Emote did not move. I tried again. Still no response. I began to be concerned.

"Emote, wake up! Remember I said when I clap my hands three times, you would wake up."

I clapped my hands louder this time and said, "Emote, can you hear me? WAKE UP!"

Emote slept on peacefully.

I was alarmed. I shook Emote gently. Even with more clapping of hands and commands to wake up . . . nothing happened.

What if she never woke up? I saw the headlines: "Coed Remains in Coma After Failed Hypnosis!"

After hours of agony, the four girls went to their rooms. I sat up all night beside the hypnotized Emote.

Every hour or so, I clapped my hands three times. The rest of the night I felt Emote's pulse and prayed, "Oh God, please have her awaken. I promise I'll never try hypnosis again if only she wakes up and is all right."

Morning finally dawned. When it was seven o'clock, I clapped my hands three more times.

Emote stirred, opened her eyes and slowly sat up. She looked around.

"What happened? Where is everybody? Why is it daylight?"

I laughed in relief and embraced the bewildered Emote. "How are you feeling?"

"I've never felt better in my life! So rested. Did I go under easy?"

"Too easy, I'm so glad you are all right, but *I'll* never be the same."

The Sinful Six were spared from any repercussions.

During the last two years of college, I went out with several students, but finally settled on one tall, slender, red-headed fellow. His father was a physician and a good friend of the Dean of Men. He had his heart set on his son becoming a doctor and tagged him with the nickname, Doc.

It seemed, though, that Doc didn't have the ability to make the grade. Doc was an excellent dancer and quite attentive, two criteria for a good date at that time

One day, I received a message to report to the Dean of Men's office the following day. I was terrified. What had I done wrong? I could not think of a thing.

The next day, I dressed as conservatively as possible and, trembling, entered the Dean's reception room. I remembered that my father knew Dean Watson very well.

His elderly secretary ushered me into the Dean's book-lined office. He rose from behind his huge mahogany desk, holding out his hand. He was a short man with small gray eyes.

"Dorothy," he said, "I'm glad to see you, but sorry it has to be for such a reason. Please be seated."

I sat on the edge of a huge leather chair and wished I was anywhere but there.

"I suppose you are wondering why I sent for you."

I nodded, unable to speak.

"I hear you are seeing a lot of Kenneth Edmonson, so I suppose you know he is flunking several of his pre-medic courses."

"No, I was not aware of that."

"Well, he is and his father is most concerned about this. As you know, no medical school will accept him with such grades. His father feels you are distracting him from his studies by seeing him every night."

I felt myself blushing in anger. I suddenly regained my voice.

"I don't know where you have received your information Dean Watson," I said, "But I have not dated *anyone* except on weekends. I promised my father I'd get good grades here and since I'm taking two majors I have to spend a lot of time studying."

"Well then, I suppose your boyfriend spends the weeknights mooning over your picture in his watch."

I became angrier and angrier. I had heard that Dean Watson had spies reporting to him, but this was the limit! Doc did have a picture of me in the back of an old fashioned watch he carried.

"I can't control what Doc does when he's not with me!" I answered.

"And I suppose you couldn't get better grades if you tried?" He felt he had played his trump card and smiled maliciously.

"No, Dean Watson," I answered, "I don't think I could because the last three semesters I've made straight A's."

Dean Watson's prominent eyes became a little more so with his obvious surprise. He cleared his throat, drummed his fingers on the desk for a few seconds and then said, "Well, see that you keep it up! You may leave now."

I didn't need a second invitation and without saying good-bye, fled back to the security of the Women's Residence Hall and the support of the Sinful Six.

Somehow or other, the gang had never approved of Doc Edmondson. They liked Emote's Fred, Ike's Earl, Nitas's Al and Frenchy's James. June did not go out regularly with any one person. She said she was "too particular." But they always criticized Doc.

I liked his sense of humor and enjoyed double dating with his roommate, who was a good looking, joking type.

One night, after a particularly uproarious night with much dancing the Charleston, the girls met in Nita's room for the customary hashing over the evening. This night they were quieter than usual with some whispering.

"What happened?" I said, "Is there something you don't want me to know about?"

More giggles and sideways glances.

Finally, Frenchy spoke up, "We did not want to tell you, but we all think you should give Doc the air."

"Why?" I asked, feeling my color rise.

"Because he's a no good, double-crossing skunk," said June.

I looked down at the fraternity pin Doc had given me the previous week in lieu of an engagement ring.

"Them's fightin' words pardner!" I quoted from our favorite western. "Put up or shut up! What's wrong with him?"

"He kissed me while we were dancing," Nita admitted. "Is that any way for an engaged man to act?"

I was crushed. In those days engagements were sacred and two-timing forbidden. I looked at Nita.

"Are you sure? Or are you just telling me this so that I'll get rid of him? I know none of you like him."

Nita snapped, "Of course I'm sure. It wasn't just a little peck on the cheek, but a real hug and a wet smack on the mouth."

I looked into Nita's sparking eyes and flushed cheeks and felt I could not blame Doc for succumbing to the charms of this little minx. Nevertheless, I decided to have it out with him.

A line of dating couples were standing two-by-two at ten o'clock Sunday night waiting for the girls to go into the Dorm. Doc and I were among them.

"I have something to ask you," I ventured.

"Yes? His superlative confidence showed through his cocky demeanor.

"Did you kiss Nita last night?"

He scowled. "How dare you ask me such a thing? We're engaged, aren't we? I wouldn't kiss anyone but you."

I saw he was lying by the way his eyes shifted away from mine. I could have tolerated the incident, but not his lying about it.

I took off his fraternity pin and handed it to him.

"Why did you do that?" he shouted.

The couples standing near us turned around.

"Because you are a liar," I shouted back.

Before I knew it, I felt a stinging blow on my cheek and Doc strode away. I had never been slapped before, not even by my parents and this was too much to bear. The girls were right. He was a skunk and I was glad to be rid of him. If we had married, he probably would have run around with anyone who would have him.

I went up to my room. No bull session tonight. I hated to face the girls and admit they had been right.

Thankfully, most of my times downstate weren't as disheartening. One of my most vivid memories and another testament to the high-jinx of the Sinful Six, also took place when the usual line-up of couples were saying good night outside the residence hall.

We all stood two-by-two like the animals going into the ark, waiting for the Saturday midnight curfew, when suddenly my friend, Kenny Schnepp, and I saw that everyone was staring up at the top of the Women's Residence Hall.

A murmur rose from the crowd as we saw a blond girl clad in a nightgown walking blithely along the parapet of the fourth floor. I gasped as I recognized the girl who could never turn down a dare — Frenchy.

Miss Blaisdell's head popped out of a third story window.

"Miss Anderson, come down immediately."

Frenchy smiled and waved as she disappeared into the skylight she had climbed through previously.

All the couples clapped.

That night the Sinful Six had an especially wild celebration, with congratulations to the intrepid Frenchy. What had Miss Blaisdell said? Was she mad? Frenchy was not talking, but smiled that enigmatic smile which infuriated all of us. Apparently her punishment had been quite severe because she did not have any dates for a month. Heaven help Miss Blaisdell when Frenchy's fertile imagination found a retaliatory measure.

It happened several months later. Miss Blaisdell had been very fond of Frenchy's long blonde hair and whenever she caught her with her braids down, she would take them in her hands and gush over them.

So one night before a weekly house meeting, Miss Blaisdell spied Frenchy sitting in the first row with her braids hanging over her shoulders.

"Oh, my dear," said Miss Blaisdell, "How I love to see such gorgeous long hair!"

She gave one of the braids a little tug and it came off in her hand! Frenchy had cut her hair that afternoon and had pinned the braids back on.

Miss Blaisdell paled, turned on her heel, and was seen no more that evening.

The rest of the Sinful Six were delighted, but I thought it was a dirty trick. I even felt a little sorry for the funny old lady, irritating though she was at times. After all, she was only trying to do her job.

The four years of premedic, scientific studies and labs, plus all the English and writing classes I could find, went by quickly. For the most part, it was a delightful experience, except for my break-up with Kenny and my enforced penalty of two months without privileges.

The Sinful Six parted with tears and promised that we would always keep in touch, which we have done throughout our lives.

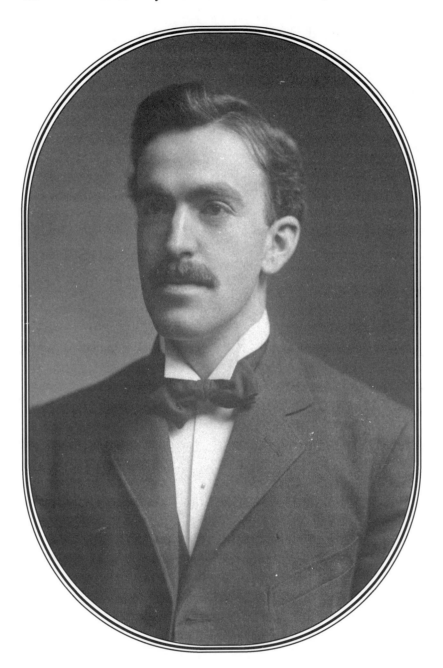

My father, William H. Welker, Phd.

MED SCHOOL

"Up and at 'em!" Father's bass voice boomed up the stairwell of our old-fashioned house in Oak Park.

I moaned and placed a pillow over my head. The first day of medical school after a sleepless night was too horrible to face.

Silence from below. If he would only go away, but I knew he would not. Head of the Department of Physiological Chemistry, Chairman of the Graduate School and Chairman of the Discipline Committee, Professor Welker was a man who always expected to be obeyed and promptly was.

"Did you hear me?" came a definitely determined voice an octave lower than before.

"Yes, I'm up," I said and tentatively put one foot onto the cold floor. I quickly pulled it back and a wave of sick apprehension engulfed me.

"What is the matter with me?" I thought. This was the moment for which I had spent four hard premedic years downstate taking a major in nutrition, so I would know how to feed my patients and another major in English so I could learn to write − a secret desire. Father would have considered it a dangerous distraction from my main purpose in life. Any hint of my desire to become an author instead of a top flight physician, not just an ordinary *Doc,* mind you, would have met with strong disapproval from his quarter.

Was that my main purpose, though? My father wanted me to

be a doctor. I was an only child and felt I had to substitute for the boy he had wanted so desperately. I hoped I could live up to his expectation. Maybe that was why I was so frightened. Who could achieve everything my father required?

I knew his students were terrified of him, especially when he walked down the hall to his first lecture of each year with his open watch in hand. At exactly eight o'clock, he snapped the watch shut and entered the lecture hall, locking the door behind him with one decisive gesture.

Nobody was ever late for Professor Welker's classes – they were absent; and three such unexcused absences caused failure for the semester. Just the sight of my father's stiff collar and black bowtie sent shivers down the students' spines.

I trembled as I hurried into the new suit I bought for the occasion. This neat little suit, a light blue wool, was a great find in Marshall Field's basement. Mother and I seldom shopped upstairs in the expensive suit department, because of Father's salary, but we always had fun any way. We were like two high school girls together.

In 1927, my new suit was the latest style, with a belted, short coat and a slightly flared skirt. Since I weighed only 95 pounds and wore a size six, I felt very trim in it. It matched my deep blue eyes and set off my luxuriant brown hair with golden-red highlights. I just had to look professional to give me confidence this first day, as I certainly wasn't feeling confident.

My mother's kind, brown eyes observed me in a most understanding way while I tried to swallow my breakfast of orange juice. I felt on the verge of tears.

"Come on. It's time," called Father from the back porch.

I snatched my purse, looked into it to see whether or not I had pencils, a pen and a small notebook. I kissed the top of Mother's head and was off.

As I ran through the grape arbor to the garage. I giggled nervously. Wouldn't it have been funny if I had been late for Professor Welker's first class? His own daughter?

However I didn't have to worry about that since, fortunately, I had taken *P. Chem* downstate. I knew if I took it in Chicago I would be criticized no matter what. A good grade would have brought forth the remark, "Well, no wonder, look whose daughter she is!" and a bad grade, "You'd think she could have done better!"

So instead, I was going to get my Master's in Protein Chemistry and would work with Father's assistant, Professor Bergheim, a round-shouldered, absent-minded darling whom I liked immediately. We were going to do a joint project on Vitamin D in white rats. But not right away, thank goodness.

We drove slowly down the middle of the boulevard toward the slum district where the old medical school was located. People had to get out of Father's way. He looked formidable sitting up straight behind the wheel of a large, ancient Buick. This car had been given to him by a doctor friend, who knew how lean his budget was in order to cover my education. Four years downstate, plus four years in medical school and two years of internship and residency took a sizeable chunk out of a professor's meager salary.

After what seemed about five hours of driving – it really was only thirty minutes – we pulled up into a public gargage. The place was dingy, the floor oil stained, smelling of machinery and dirty mechanics. Medical school could not be worse than this!

My father was methodically racing the engine for a few seconds. He climbed out of the car and smiled at me, his deep blue eyes kindly.

I tried to smile back.

"Well, today's the start of the race, isn't it?"

I shivered. I hoped he had not noticed. "Yes, I'm thrilled about it."

"It's a big undertaking," he said, waving to the garage man. "But soon the four years will have gone by quickly."

I could not imagine it. Those four years loomed ahead interminably, filled with endless obstacles. I hinted as much.

Father laughed heartily.

"Many other people have gone through this and were none the worse."

"But girls?" I wondered out loud.

"Dorothy," he answered seriously, "Forget about that part of it. Many doctors advise their daughters against studying medicine, but I could not see it that way with *you*."

This rare compliment delighted me. We walked along the grimy street in the direction of the medical school.

"I thought," he continued, "that you could immerse your inherent feminine timidity in the conscientious application to your work. I know you will prove my theory is correct."

I smiled.

Suddenly, the once distant structure loomed up in front of us looking not nearly as fearsome as I had remembered it from childhood visits to the place. It was a four story, dirty, red brick building with stains of rain water mixed with soot running down from the broken eaves.

In front of the medical building, there were many soapstone steps worn into low curves by the tred of hundreds of medical students. I wondered if any of those footsteps had been as halting as mine.

Inside the widely swinging front doors, was a hodgepodge of strange faces. I noticed that most of them were moustached. Did they feel that a hairy upper lip made them look more mature? They all seemed greatly impressed with the seriousness of their profession. They walked importantly, as though they were saying to themselves, "We are going to be doctors."

I did not like this at all. I felt many people staring at me and even heard, "That's Professor Welker and his daughter."

Why, it was as bad as it was downstate with its gossiping, peering and jabbering!

Father walked ahead into the Registrar's office. There was deference from all sides and more restrained curiosity. I was introduced to a capable looking secretary and a piquant, Irish cashier. Father wrote a check for my registration fee.

Should I back out now, before it was too late? I wondered, but was stopped by the awesome presence of my father.

The door opened and the very serious Registrar of the school entered with pomposity. I had met him at numerous social functions.

"Well, well, well! What have we here? A new student?"

I smiled politely, I hoped, and we exchanged a few brief comments.

He dismissed me with, "Run right along, my dear." he said, patting my hand in a paternal gesture. "Pick up your schedule in my office. Come in to see me later if you get into any trouble."

"Nice man," I thought, "Even though somewhat affected." I liked him in spite of his fake English accent.

Father then left me and I felt that his receding figure took with him all connection with my past life.

I went into the corridor to be immediately engulfed by a shouting mob which was moving violently toward the stairs. Small students, tall students, an occasional fat student, many thin students, gesticulating, examining bulletin boards, slapping each others backs somewhat as they had done downstate, but more fiercely and with an intense preoccupation with their future careers . . . and no girls around.

I would find out that this 1929 Freshman Class of one hundred and eighty-five medical students was comprised of nearly all men and only four women. We four were lucky to have been there at all. Women were not welcomed in medical schools throughout the country. In fact, Northwestern University refused to accept women at all for many more years.

I worked my way through the mass of bodies, leaving a little path of silence behind. I walked up four flights of worn, wooden stairs and then through a dark corridor which harbored a very odd odor and into an ancient gymnasium.

Pygmied under high wooden rafters were many camp chairs set around rickety tables. Spread over the whole was a rather bewildered looking crowd of students. Here and there was a familiar face from my premedic classes, but most of the men were strangers, many of them homely and studious looking.

I looked around eagerly in order to find any other girls. I saw one very square shaped, mannish looking one with thick glasses and flat shoes, another slender, slightly stooped, older woman and then – wonder of wonders – a pretty, pink cheeked, little blonde with big, startled blue eyes. She was accompanied by two tall, handsome men who apparently were laughing at her fears.

Barbara Benda smiled at my astonishment. "I kept it a secret for the last year downstate so that you'd be surprised to see me here." I held out my hand with good comradeship as we renewed a rather desultory acquaintance of our premedic days. Barbara's smile was guarded as though she were measuring a possible opponent.

Beneath the small talk of registration and section, putting us into groups of fifteen to thirty students, an old conundrum was renewed in my mind. Why could women not accept each other as men did? Why were they, except for a few, always on the alert, watching, covering, fencing? My open-heartedness had received many a rebuff, because I could not assume that attitude toward acquaintances.

Here again, I felt a feminine wariness in Barbara which was so foreign to my nature.

A senior medical student came up, very much the professional woman in a tailored suit and a severe hat. Barb and I exchanged a small, wordless, eye comment on her mannishness before she was upon us.

"How are you girls getting on?" she asked. I'm Miss Gladys Washburn," she introduced herself in a school teacherish manner, as though at any moment she would ask us to name the boundaries of Asia or describe the posterior triangle of the neck.

We murmured the usual meaningless responses to questions which are really not supposed to be answered, or if they are answered, are not listened to.

"I suppose you have arranged for your partners," Miss Washburn said with her firm lips, but her eyes dictated, *If you haven't done so, you'd better get on with it!*

I felt a little uneasy at the strangeness of it all.

Then Miss Washburn nodded briskly, saying, "If there's anything I can do, let me know." She turned quickly and was out of the room in three strides.

Several of the men smiled condescendingly and I flushed at their remark, "She's a typical *Hen Medic.*"

Barbara was a relief standing there, her blue eyes wide with wonder. "Hen Medic?" She had never heard the term.

"Oh, that's just a nasty name a lot of med students use for women doctors. I've always hated it," I remarked.

"So do I," agreed Barbara.

"It's wonderful to have you here," I sighed with relief.

Barbara looked at the tallest of her two companions and blushed, "Well, I did promise Ty I'd be his anatomy lab partner," she said, "but if you'd rather that I'd be yours, I can always change."

I shook my head, "I'll find someone else," I told her, but I was a little annoyed.

Just then Kenny Schnepp, a friend I had dated quite a few times downstate, came to my rescue. Though I'd been expecting him, he was late as usual and looking as nonchalant and incorrigible as ever.

"Did I hear that you need an anatomy lab partner? Glad to oblige."

I agreed doubtfully. He had a reputation for being a little wild, although he had been gentlemanly on our dates. I could not imagine dissecting cadavers with him, but for that matter, I could not imagine dissecting a cadaver with anyone at all. Oh well, one hurdle at a time.

"Did you get my schedule?" he asked.

I had it, as usual, spoiling him.

A stubby, rotund, middle-aged man was rapping on the podium for attention. The noisy group quieted down.

"Ladies and Gentlemen," he said stiffly, "I am Professor Davis, your Dean. That is, Dean of the College of Medicine. Welcome to the College. Classes start today. All who have not pre-registered, go to the registration office. The remainder of you, pick up your schedules here," he pointed to a pile of envelopes on the podium and left.

"Jolly chap, isn't he?" grinned Kenny in his usual sardonic style.

I went to my first class, Histology. It was a gloomy, dusty lab with long narrow tables and high stools to sit on while viewing slides through a microscope. Two white-coated instructors showed the thirty students of Section Three to their places.

The young instructors did not bother to introduce themselves. I learned later that histology was part of the Department of Anatomy and that these minor teaching jobs were often delegated to men working their way through medical school, therefore of little importance in the hierarchy.

"Your next class will be day after tomorrow," our instructor spoke quickly. "Be sure to bring your microscopes. We will furnish the slides. You will also need a set of colored drawing pencils and a five by eight, unlined notebook with a hard cover. You will be asked to copy accurately and in detail the tissue assigned to you."

The students groaned.

A small smile lifted the corners of the instructor's mouth. "Your text is Berger's Histology. You may leave now."

I consulted my schedule. Nothing more until after lunch. I suddenly realized I was hungry. I asked Barbara, "How about going for a snack, if you can pry yourself from your admirers?"

We crossed Harrison Street to the *Greeks*, a customary gathering place of students, interns and residents. It was jammed with noisy, loud talking men.

Barbara was babbling as was her tendency. Her father had bought her a shiny, new, binocular microscope, with three lenses, which she described in detail.

I thought ruefully of the ancient brass microscope which my father had bought for me from one of his graduate students. There were many such short cuts that had to be made, I knew, but nevertheless I resented them. I felt like an ungrateful wretch, but I couldn't help it. It was great that my father had managed to send me at all, I supposed.

We finished lunch and then it was time to face one of the courses I dreaded most – Anatomy.

Professor Kitchner, head of the Anatomy Department, was fortyish, tall, lean and intense. He was well known for his exquisite drawings on the blackboard. Professor Kitchner was busily engaged in making such a multi-colored work of art when I entered the room. I gasped at the sight. He was drawing meticulous diagrams with both hands, simultaneously and equally well. Much to my disappointment, he stopped this amazing feat and turned around to call the roll, making note of any absentees. His speech was clipped and precise.

"The Anatomy course consists of two semesters of dissecting a cadaver, one half of which each of you will be responsible for and also two semesters of didactic lectures with theoretical and practical tests covering them. You will be required to know the names, origins, insertions and functions of all main muscles; names of all bones; names, distributions and functions of main nerves, including cranial nerves; and the site of all organs, plus their blood and nerve supply. Next year, in Neurology, you will study the brain in detail."

After giving the students their assignment, Dr. Kitchner dismissed them with a pleasant nod.

I went slowly up to Father's office on the second floor. I felt overwhelmed with all that was expected of me but I knew I could never let him know this. He had been so proud of all of my A's downstate and I couldn't let him down now.

He was smoking his pipe and reading a scientific journal at his roll top desk. He smiled when I came in.

"Well *Pickles*, how did it go?" He only used this silly nickname when he was feeling particularly fond of me.

"Oh, okay I guess. I saw the two handed wonder drawing cross-sections of the spinal cord on the board in anatomy."

He snorted with delight. He was not too fond of Professor Kitchner's exhibitionism, as he called it, so he liked my description of him.

"Ready to go home?" I hoped he was. I wanted to get away from all of these challenges.

I fell asleep that night impatiently awaiting the second day and wondering whether this strange hold the idea of a medical career had on me would become an actuality, especially now that the study of medicine hovered over me. My dreams were a jumble of steel lockers, fee slips, schedules and mustachioed freshman peering at me and yelling, "Hen medic."

Next morning, I put on my feathered mules and ran to the window to see what kind of a day it was. It was raining in great sheets, making a white flurry in the bird bath, drenching the cherry tree, the grape arbor and sinking my hopes of wearing my new suit for fear it would be water-spotted.

I shivered, closing the window with a bang. I would have laughed at anyone who told me I was superstitious, but the weather seemed an omen of discouragement and failure.

My mood lightened as Mother's happy voice called me to breakfast. That sound always helped things and it *was* a great relief to be home again, looking out at the familiar back yard, even though, at the moment, it was soaked with rain.

My four pre-medic years had been lots of fun, at times, with amusing dates, but troublesome at others, as when I'd had to break my engagement. Now, I felt that my little sailboat of an education had entered a calm, safe harbor, at least temporarily. I hurried down to my mother's home-cooked breakfast.

What a complete contrast my parents were. Father was blue

eyed, dignified, strong-willed and competent, not only in chemistry, medicine and engineering; but in woodworking, fly tying and repairing household equipment in his complete workshop in the basement.

Mother, on the other hand, was frail and lovely with large brown eyes and soft dark hair fastened straight back into a small bun at the nap of her neck. She spoke quietly, but everything she said made sense. She seldom thought of herself and her greatest happiness lay in helping others. Yet, there was nothing martyr-like about her for she had a marvelous sense of humor and made little jokes, many of them at her own expense.

She was loving, young at heart and a delightful companion for me. She would race me to the mailbox like a teenager and she taught me how to sit a horse without any daylight showing between me and the saddle. She had shocked the small Pennsylvania Dutch community where she had been brought up by being the first horsewoman to give up the side saddle and ride astride.

Mother had advised me, "Don't pay attention to what people say about you, as long as you know in your heart that what you are doing is right."

Mother never preached unwanted advice to me and I was grateful for that. So many of my peers complained that their parents and grandparents went on endlessly about the "shoulds" and "should nots" of their actions. They resented being "treated like children."

So I went on to my second year of medical school gratefully unencumbered by all sorts of unwanted advice.

Anatomy lab was on the fourth floor of the Dental Building. It, like the old Medical Building, was circa 1888 and smelled of decay and mold. The climb up the steep wooden stairs made me breathless. It was very hot and each ascending floor seemed ten degrees hotter than the last. I worried what I would find up there. I'd heard weird tales about the anatomy lab from upper classmen who took delight in frightening freshmen.

Dozens of students huddled on the fourth floor landing. A little, strutting instructor with thinning gray hair and a Russian sounding accent greeted us with a sadistic smile.

"Ladies and gentlemen, your cadavers await you. Out of courtesy to our four females, we will allow them to go first. Walk down the aisle and choose your patient. I hope you have your dissecting sets with you." He opened the door.

I glanced in apprehensively. Rows and rows of still figures wrapped in layers of cheesecloth lay on tables on each side of a wide aisle at the far end of which were six narrow, dirt encrusted windows.

Barbara, Miriam, Denise and I started our long, hesitant walk between the white, still figures. I remembered I had been told to pick a lean cadaver so that I would not have to cut through an inch or two of fat. But how could I tell about the cadaver under all those layers of cheesecloth?

"I guess we'll just have to pinch them," said Miriam matter of factly and doing just that. She finally found her victim and Denise stayed with her as her partner.

Barbara and I shuddered and kept walking toward the far distant window. A strong smell of formaldehyde mixed with the sweetish smell of decay engulfed us, I felt nauseated.

The boys left behind yelled, "Hurry up!" They were anxious to pick out the man or woman they would examine for the next two semesters.

Barbara and I reached the end of the rows. It was now or never. Barbara turned to the figure on the left and I reached out tentatively to touch the cadaver on the right. I knew I had to feel for good muscles, but I shrank from the task. I looked across at Barbara who smiled encouragingly. She liked my choice.

I reached my hand out once more, grasped the cadaver's arm and nearly fainted. It was WARM! It took me several minutes to realize the arm was room temperature and that my hand was ice cold. Could there be anything worse than this?

The boys came crowding in and I was glad when Kenny

found me and approved my choice of cadaver, which looked like a sailor with large tattoo marks on his arms and chest. He was young, hairy and muscular. We named him Barnacle Bill and Kenny carefully removed his tattoos as souvenirs. I thought, *How could he?*

I wondered what happened to the sailor. He must have had a violent death to die so young and unemaciated. As we unwrapped the upper part of his body, which we would work on the first semester, we could find no bullet marks. It was very exciting now that the first shock was over. We pretended that we were pathologists doing an autopsy on a puzzling case.

The little instructor suddenly appeared at our table.

"Do the lower arms and hands first, *doctors*," he said sarcastically. "Every muscle must be cleanly dissected so that you can demonstrate the origins and insertions of each one." He noticed the surgical gloves that I was wearing, not a requirement, or even commonly used then.

"Afraid to get your hands dirty? Such a lady! Whoever told you, you could be a doctor?"

I looked straight into his squinty little eyes. "My father, Professor Welker," I told him, matter of factly.

Dr. Weinstein appeared puzzled and then suddenly enlightened and embarrassed. He lowered his head and sidled away crab-like.

"That's telling him!" said Kenny, going back to his dissection. "He's a real creep."

I laughed. I had won my first encounter with woman doctor prejudice. I knew I would meet up with much of this attitude in the future and somehow it gave me the courage to go on. Also, the amused expression in Kenny's kind, hazel eyes helped.

Kenny never took anything too seriously, except his deep desire to be a surgeon. He had been trained to be a concert pianist and the dexterity of his long fingers was apparent in the ease with which he dissected even the tiniest nerve fibers. His father had discouraged him from going to Europe to continue his musical studies, so Kenny turned to his next goal, medicine. When we were dating in Urbana-Champaign, Kenny had persuaded me to watch an operation. We drove up to Oak Park in his gorgeous, new, lemon-yellow Packard convertible, the envy of all the girls in my dormitory. We stayed at my house on Friday night and drove down early the next morning to Augustana Hospital to view a thyroidectomy by the great thyroid surgeon, Dr Percy. Kenny had an intern friend who helped us crash the gate. We climbed up into the high balcony over looking the operating pit.

I had heard about the students fainting at the first operation, so I was very proud of feeling fine as I looked at the gaping wound in the patient's neck. It was almost eight inches across and surrounded by dozens of shining, stainless steel hemostats used to stop the bleeding. I grasped the bar in front of me and leaned in for a closer look.

Kenny was engrossed in the technique of the operation, explaining it to me every step of the way. "See how carefully Dr. Percy is dissecting out the thyroid gland and leaving the parathyroids intact. If he removed them, the patient might have convulsions due to interference with her calcium metabolism. Also, he must be careful not to cut either one of the recurrent laryngeal nerves or she would not be able to speak." He had been reading surgery articles for the last two years.

I tried to see over the shoulders of the residents assisting Dr. Percy, but all I could see was the huge red hole in the patient's neck. Thank goodness for general anesthesia, I thought.

Then Dr. Percy's voice rose to question the patient, "How do you feel?"

I thought, The patient is asleep. How can she hear him? But the woman could, because she answered, "Just fine, doctor."

It was too much for me. I felt very warm and my hands and feet prickled. The next thing I knew, I woke up flat on my back in the men's room with Kenny pouring a glass of water on my face.

"What happened?" I asked weakly.

"You fainted, you chicken you," said Kenny, chuckling gleefully. "Didn't you know the whole operation was done under local?"

I sat up, patted the water from my face and sighed.

"Oh Kenny, I'll never be a doctor!"

Now here I was, one year later, ready to cut into my first cadaver with Kenny at my side once again and I'd be darned if I was going to faint this time.

I made it through that first day and many more thereafter.

After a summer vacation, the class of 1931 congregated in the gymnasium the way they had the previous year, only this time there were no frightened faces. There is nothing more confident than a sophomore medical student. Never in our entire careers would we think we knew so much. The honorary title of Doctor, which we were given facetiously by our teachers, was taken seriously and we thought we knew all the answers.

"The weak-kneed ones," as my father called them, had been weeded out. Over fifteen percent of the class were forced to seek less demanding occupations and the remainder of the class was proud to have survived. We were now starting the first semester of our second year of medical school. The year was 1929.

Our cadavers had been dissected down to the muscles. All the organs had been removed and examined carefully. When Kenny and I came to Barnacle Bill's heart, we made an exciting discovery. The embalming fluid leaked out of a tear about an inch long in one of the heart chambers; the right ventricle. This clay-like pink material had spilled out into the entire mediastinum, the cavity in which the heart lay like a bell in its cupola. Only this bell did not chime anymore because some assailant's knife had silenced it forever. The two amateur pathologists had discovered the cause of the death of Barnacle Bill, so young and so handsome.

"I'm sure he got into a fight over some dame," said Kenny with a significant gleam in his eyes.

"Why do you think everything violent has to be connected with a woman?" I asked, industriously removing the mass of embalming fluid while giving a sidewise, disgusted glance at two men at the next table who were happily munching candy bars while carrying on their dissection.

"Because it usually is," answered Kenny in his sardonic way.

He really looked like a satyr I thought, with his slanted eyebrows and slightly pointed ears.

For several months he had assiduously pursued me with a semi-comic imitation of a man in love. I thought he could never be serious about affairs of the heart and that's why I just couldn't get involved emotionally with him.

He was not used to being refused, so my brushing aside of his invitations to see his *pad* made me all the more appealing to him.

Instead of a romantic entanglement, we had great times attending jazz concerts, fraternity dances, plays, movies and listening to Glen Miller and Duke Ellington records.

Kenny played jazz piano very well and was in demand for fraternity parties. I used to sit on the piano bench beside him, entranced by the dexterity of his flying fingers.

My father scornfully called his performances, "Saloon piano playing," but how did Father know since he had never entered a saloon or tavern? I wondered.

Of course, it did seem a waste of time and talent when Kenny had practiced so long and hard on his classical concerts. But that was how some parents were, always interfering.

I remembered how desperately I had wanted to go on tour with my dance group. I had timorously entered Father's office one spring vacation and asked permission to go to South America the coming summer of my junior year downstate.

He puffed meditatively on his pipe for several minutes and then said, "Well Dorothy, now is the time to make up your mind whether you want to be a dancer or a doctor. If you choose dancing you will be through by the time you are thirty-five, but if you choose medicine you will just be starting, with a whole life of service ahead of you at that age. Think it over," he admonished and dismissed me with a definitive gesture.

I was deeply disappointed and had to tell my dance instructor that the answer was, "No," as none of the group could go without their parents' permission. I brooded about it all summer, but in the fall had to accept the logic of his suggestion. Still, whenever I attended a ballet or even heard the familiar strains of the overtures to Les Sylphides and of the Nutcracker Suite, my heart gave a little leap of recognition and regret.

I attended every performance I could of good ballet companies and, while sitting in the first row of the balcony of Orchestral Hall, I was transported onto the stage in the person of a prima ballerina like Doniliva, dancing a pas de deux with Frederick Franklin. Of course, I would have been just a member of the corp de ballet, but I thought when I fantasized, I might as well fantasize being at the top. So for each two or three hours of a performance, I was delighted, transported from my medical studies for these brief, idyllic interludes.

Second year medical school was much like the first only with different scientific subjects; Neurology, Pharmacy, Bacteriology and Physiology. I was not as terrified of going to school each day, except for taking examinations, which really upset me.

One day, while I was worrying over the exact answer to a question, my Bacteriology professor, Dr. Barton, bent over me and said, "Why do you take your exams so seriously? It is not the end of the world, you know."

"It would be for me if I failed."

He laughed, "Relax. Live a little. You are young and pretty. Enjoy yourself. Don't worry so much!"

I looked at him as he strolled away. That was easy enough for him to say. While Dr. Barton had been an undergraduate student downstate, he had discovered a method of making the cotton fibers of feminine hygiene pads much more absorbent of liquids. With the proceeds of a patent sold to a manufacturer of this product and wise investments of the same, he was financially set for life.

However, I did feel more calm and wrote a good examination.

Things were going better than I had expected, except for Physiology. It was absolute torture to go to the laboratory and operate on living dogs. It was true that they were anesthetized but when I walked over to my operating table and saw a cute, little, shaggy terrier on its back with its four paws restrained by leather thongs, I almost decided to give up medical school.

I always loved animals, almost as much as people, because they seemed so appealing and helpless and because they were grateful for any affection I gave them. I had always owned a dog and had felt bereft when my last one, a Belgian Shepherd, had been poisoned by a neighbor just a few weeks previously.

Now to have to operate on a pretty, little dog was too terrible to attempt. I knew that students had to learn to handle tissue, to incise, to tie off blood vessels so that they could do the same to their human patients, but I thought there should be a better way to learn.

My gentle, old Physiology professor noticed that I was just standing beside Kenny while he was blissfully operating without any help from me.

"Dorothy dear, you'd better come into my office for a few minutes," he said softly, taking my arm. I came with him gratefully, leaving the chamber of horrors.

He sat down beside me on his couch in the cheerful space, half sitting room and half office. We were old friends since my parents and I had often visited him and his invalid wife, who was badly incapacitated with rheumatoid arthritis.

"Oh, Dr. Darcy, how can you stand working with those poor dogs, day after day?"

"Now Dorothy, I know how you feel, brought up in a sheltered environment away from the realities of life, but if you are determined to be a doctor you must learn to accept all kinds of unpleasant experiences."

"I can deal with people suffering, but I can't stand hurting animals. It's because I can't *explain* to them why they are in pain and why I must be so cruel."

"My dear," he said sadly, "these animals are not feeling any pain. They are anesthetized and will be until the operations are over when they will be sacrificed."

"Sacrificed? What does that mean?"

"We believe that they must not suffer so we pour ether down their throats. They die without waking up. Now do you feel a little better?" His gray eyes, surrounded with smile wrinkles, looked deeply into mine.

I did feel a little better and tried to smile back.

"How will you ever be a good intern and resident, helping in the operating room if you don't develop your primary skills now? You will see a heart pumping blood and peristaltic waves going through the stomach and intestines of these canines just as you will see in humans. You will learn how to handle a liver gently so as not to damage it. You will locate a spleen tucked away under the ribs on the left side and know how to remove it without too much bleeding. You cannot practice on humans and I'm sure you would not want to."

He patted my ice cold hands clasped tightly in my lap. He really was kind and reassuring and I appreciated it, but I felt I'd had enough of that day.

"Do you mind if I go home now?" I asked quietly.

He smiled, "If you like, but I want to see you here at the next lab session for sure."

I promised and left, as usual heading for Father's office, my refuge whenever I was troubled. There he was, stern, rock-like, that eternally smoking pipe protruding from his mouth.

"Through so soon?" he asked, noticing, I'm sure, how pale and shaken I looked.

"I'm through, but the class isn't."

"Want to go home, now?"

"Oh yes." I was grateful there were no more questions.

"Well, let's go," he said, matter-of-factly and we were off.

Although Father held high expectations of me, he never pushed me beyond my limits. I will always be grateful for his firm, but kind, handling of my sensitivity.

Soon, the two didactic years were over and I was glad of that, especially since I was through with the horrors of Physiology. Now, in the following two clinical years, would come application of all that I had learned in my pre-clinical studies. I looked forward to that.

GETTING INTO THE THICK OF IT

Part of the surgical course requirement was for the students to attend the surgical outpatient clinic. The Third Section was particularly fortunate in having the head of the department, Dr. Linden Seed, as their professor. To have the head of the department as instructor was a rare occurrence, but necessitated in this case, because the regular instructor was ill.

This tall and angular, acrid man was an excellent teacher, although his method of driving facts home often left lasting scars.

At our first session, he gave us a few caustic remarks: "This is not going to be easy. I am going to drill some important facts into your heads and I expect them to remain there. Also some of the patients I will show you will be ugly sights and many of them won't smell too pleasant either. I don't want any of you fainting. If you do, I'll stand you on your heads." He glared at each student as though he meant it. I remembered how I had fainted at seeing my first operation and prayed I would not do it again.

The first few sessions went very well and our section learned many important facts.

However, on the third day, the twenty students of Section Three were crowded into a small examining room around a twelve-year-old boy with a bull neck. He had tuberculous cervical lymph adenitis, an infection of the lymph nodes of the neck with dozens of draining sinuses. Horrible smelling pus was oozing out of many of the holes and the room was permeated with this stench.

Dr. Seed was discussing the way the infection had started and traveled through the body when, all at once, his voice seemed far away to me. I felt very warm and my fingers tingled – both tell-tale signs. I pushed past my classmates, heading for the door. I was not going to be stood on my head!

When I reached the hall I still felt giddy so I headed blindly for the elevator, managing to get safely inside before I fell flat on the floor. The elevator rose to the second floor where Father's lab was situated.

I awoke stretched out on one of his laboratory stands surrounded by Bunsen burners and all kinds of beakers and bottles. But I did not pay too much attention to them because just a few inches away from my face, were the bespectacled, frog-like features of Dr. Isadore Press. He had recognized me in the elevator and had dragged me into Father's lab where he had laid me out on the chemistry slab.

I thought, "This is what hell must be like with the devil peering down at you!"

Dr. Press was laughing, "So you've decided to return to the land of the living. Welcome back. I thought you were gone for good. What happened to you?"

I shook my head and sat up gingerly. I was not going to tell this tormentor of women medical students what his colleague in crime, Dr. Seed, had done to me. It would give him too much satisfaction.

I slid off the table and headed for my usual sanctuary, Father's office. Dr. Press trailed behind and followed me in.

"I found her conked out in the elevator," he said importantly. "This is what happens when we allow females into medical schools."

Father lead me to a chair because I still looked shaky.

He dismissed Isadore with a curt nod and evidently did not

consider his remark worth answering.

When he left, he said, "Pay no attention to him or to Dr. Seed. They are in the minority. Most of the members of the medical staff are gentlemen and are glad to have women here. You will find that to be true throughout medical school and your internship and residency."

However, there were several more unpleasant incidents still to come. Dr. Seed was not through with me yet.

I was horrified when I received a "C" on my semi-final examination in Surgery. I knew I had answered all the questions correctly, so I fretted over it for several days before gathering enough courage to talk to Dr. Seed about it. I stood by his desk until the last curious member of the class had left.

"Yes?" he asked brusquely.

"I wonder what I got wrong on my exam." I asked.

Dr. Seed smiled smugly, "I haven't the least idea."

"Did someone else correct my paper?"

"No, I always read all of the exams except those of the women. I give them all C's."

I gasped, "Why?"

"Well, the dumb ones flunk out of medical school anyhow and the bright ones get married and never practice medicine. It's just a waste of time."

I realized it would not do any good to argue with him, but I had to get in one parting shot.

"Well, I intend to pass every course and hopefully make A.O.A. (honorary medical society) and I don't want a "C" in a large course like Surgery to stand in my way. I am going to take this examination for re-evaluation to Dean Watson."

Dr. Seed grabbed the paper out of my hand and mumbled, "I'll read it this time."

My father approved of my action and told me about a run-in he had with Dr. Seed some time before.

They were fishing on Fox Lake during a faculty excursion day. My father was a skilled fly fisherman who considered fishing with live bait an abomination.

Dr. Seed dug a can full of worms and hid it under the seat of the small boat that my father was rowing. They were almost at the propitious spot, when Father scooped the can up and threw it overboard.

Dr. Seed demanded, "What the hell do you think you are doing? I spent a whole hour digging up those worms!"

Father replied innocently, "Oh, were those worms? I just thought it was a dirty old can cluttering up the boat."

It wasn't until Father told me that story that I realized, where Dr. Seed was concerned, I had two strikes against me; I was a woman and I was Professor Welker's daughter.

Years later, I would sit next to Dr. Seed at a faculty dinner honoring my father for his twenty-five years as Head of the Physiological Chemistry Department. It was a fun evening, patterned on the college roast traditions.

I could not resist roasting Dr. Seed a bit myself.

"Do you remember when you said that all dumb female medical students flunked out and all the bright ones get married and give up their practices?"

He nodded.

"Well, here I am, Dr. Seed, with a busy practice, a husband and two children. What do you have to say about your theory now?"

He grinned at me wickedly and answered, "Why aren't you home taking care of your children?"

It seemed I'd never win against that man. He always had to have the last word.

My next clerkship after surgery was Obstetrics. It was fascinating to me, but a little terrifying as well. I was teamed with another medical student and a nurse. We were sent out into the slums to deliver a baby. Conditions were primitive, to say the least. We were equipped with a large bag of sterile instruments and medications, including antiseptics – but no antibiotics, because none had been discovered by this time.

We had been instructed on the technique of bringing a human being into the world, but with no practical experience, these instructions meant very little. It is true, an obstetrical resident was on call if we had any difficulty in the delivery, but he was way back at the Illinois Research Hospital which was many miles away. I shuddered when I thought of all the possibilities. I asked my partner, a tall, pleasant, young medical student whether he felt the least bit nervous.

Ernest Otto van der Aue smiled and said, "Not really. They try to pick a multipara, a woman who has had several babies previously without complications, so she probably could have this one without our help."

We were splashing through the dirty slush on the West Side of Chicago, one of the poorest sections in town. The patient lived five flights up so we were winded when we arrived at the cracked wooden door. No bell, so we knocked. After a short wait, the door opened and there stood an old white woman with a very black two-year-old child by her side.

"Are you the doctors? We've been waiting a long time," she said contentiously. "Come here Dan!" She dragged at the boy's arm. He whimpered.

"Are you the baby sitter?" I asked, trying to get my bearings.

The woman gave a scornful laugh, "Hell no. I'm the grandmother!" She dared me to make some sign of surprise.

Van and I went past her into the bedroom from which poignant wails were coming every three minutes.

A nurse rose from a chair by the bedside. She had spread newspapers under the patient, since they were cleaner than the sheets on which the woman was lying.

A nice looking, mulatto man of about twenty-four years, was holding another black child by the hand. He was the son of the woman who met us at the door.

His greeting was more civil than his mother's had been. "I'm so glad you've arrived. I think my wife is about due."

We scrubbed in the tiny kitchen and I was glad we had

brought clean soap and towels with us. We put on sterile gowns, masks and gloves and went to work. In about ten minutes, a healthy little infant made her appearance. We tied the cord with sterile white tape and then delivered the placenta.

The nurse wrapped the baby in a warm blanket and handed it to the mother. She held it close, accepting her little infant. The father stretched out his arms and held the baby tenderly. I told him it was a girl.

He looked very sad. "I thought you'd be happy to get a girl after four boys," I mentioned, looking at four little boy faces crowding around the baby.

The father sighed, "Boys are OK, but little girls are special. How can I buy her the pretty dresses and other nice things she should have?"

He was a handsome man, with beautiful cafe-au-lait colored skin and Jamaican features. His shoulders drooped slightly as he left the room and I wanted to give him some encouraging words, but the situation looked so hopeless that I did not know how to reassure him.

I asked the mother, "What are you going to name her?" The woman shook her head. She did not know.

I followed the husband into the bare living room. "What are you going to call your daughter?"

"You name her, Doctor. You probably have named lots of babies."

I was silent. I could not tell him that this was my first delivery, then, all at once, I had an idea! "This is Valentine's Day, isn't it?" I asked.

Years later, I would wonder whatever became of the cute, little, black girl named Valentine and her sad father.

After that first delivery, my obstetrical clerkship was upon me before I knew it. In clerkships, we gained practical experience in each speciality. My Internal Medicine clerkship had been very interesting and educational, but I dreaded this OB clerkship.

I had spent a restless night trying to sleep in the nurses' dressing room just off the OB ward. I was worrying about my patient in labor. One of the residents told me that I had to deliver ten patients myself without any help and I was not looking forward to it. This was my first, not counting the home delivery of Valentine.

The corridor was long, white and cold. I was shaking in my white, intern's uniform, bought for this occasion. I thought, "That poor woman. She must be suffering terribly. What if she bleeds? What if the baby is a breech – coming bottom first instead of head first? What will I do?"

After scrubbing, I arrived at the delivery room door. I pushed it open with my elbow, dreading to see the torment that my first patient was in.

There she lay, or rather *rested* on her side, her elbow propped on the delivery table, her chin snuggled comfortably in her palm.

"How are you feeling?" I asked anxiously while donning my sterile cap, mask, gown and gloves.

"I'm just fine!" The big woman grinned at me, noticing how thin and pale I was. "By the looks of things, I'm feeling better than you are , honey, Am I your first patient?"

"My second."

"Don't worry, I'll tell you what to do. I know all about it. I've had seven kids before this one."

All at once the humor of the situation hit me and I giggled. "OK, let's go!"

The delivery went so smoothly that the resident was surprised when he sauntered in a half-hour later.

The infant, all eight pounds of him, was crying lustily. He was wrapped up and warm. The cord was tied, the placenta delivered and the mother smiled broadly.   "The doctor did just fine!" she told the residents. "She'll be OK."

I went down the corridor to my room thanking God for the wonderful experience of birth which I had witnessed. What a happy introduction to OB! I wished all my patients would be as friendly and cooperative as Zarah Moon had been, but I was afraid it was an impossible dream, and it was.

The remainder of my OB clerkship was quite uneven, with patients of all ages, sizes and conditions. The only common demoninator was the place where the deliveries occurred on the Obstetrical Floor of the University of Illinois Research Hospital.

The patients that troubled me the most were the youngest ones, many of whom were no more than twelve to fourteen years of age. I could hardly stand watching their tortured faces or hearing their pitiful cries. They were so innocent and childish. The memory of those *babies having babies* has haunted me ever since.

I survived my OB clerkship and found that one of the most interesting specialties I encountered in my third year was Ear, Nose and Throat. The clinical lectures were fascinating, but unfortunately, one of my most vivid memories associated with that speciality is an unpleasant one.

The most interesting of all the clinical lectures the third year students had were those of Ear, Nose and Throat. The professor and head of the department was a brilliant, short, wiry man who liked to start his lectures with slightly off-color jokes.

The four girls sat in the front row because we objected to the boys turning around and looking at us when we were embarrassed by the lurid punch lines. Even then, we could feel the backs of our necks get red under the scrutiny of hundreds of pairs of eyes. It was one of the few times that I minded being a woman.

Dr. Landau also liked to demonstrate what he was lecturing on by bringing one of the students up in front of the class and showing off a particular abnormality. I did not know that soon I would be the victim in front of the class. It was a day when Dr. Landau was discussing the tongue. He told everyone to stick out his or her tongue and went up and down the aisles examining each one with his flashlight.

He had one student come up to the front of the class as an

awful example of a tongue "with a coat and vest" on it as a result of a hangover and another boy who had a striated tongue like hills and valleys called a "geographic tongue."

Then he asked me to come to the front of the class and stick out my tongue. I knew it was different than all the rest because it had deep crevasses in it, a congenital defect.

Dr. Landau was in his element, speaking as though he were a barker at a sideshow in the circus. "Now here is a young lady with a most interesting tongue. Her mother probably did not get proper nourishment during her pregnancy so that the sections forming the tongue did not unite completely. It has many rugae in it so it's called 'scrotal tongue'. Come up and examine it."

There erupted much laughter from the class and I was filled with embarrassment and confusion. I wanted to go back to my seat but was surrounded with delighted classmates peering at my peculiar tongue and making all manner of wise cracks.

I was mortified. I wanted to kick them in the shins and was sorely tempted to tell them what I had told previous curious acquaintances when they had asked me how I had developed those cracks in my tongue; that every time I told a lie my father had taken out his pocket knife and made a cut in my tongue. I was amazed when they believed me!

Years later when I made house calls on Dr. Landau's twin grandchildren I recalled the incident somewhat to his embarrassment.

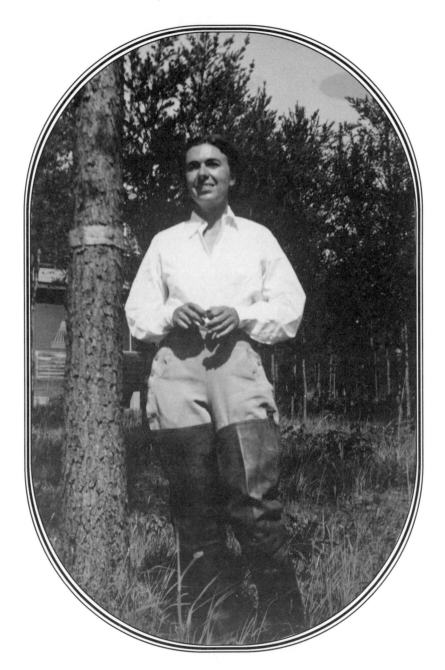

At my beloved Lake Gilmore

A DANGEROUS ROMANCE

One of the clerkships that students looked forward to was a two-week stay in the Municipal Tuberculosis Sanitarium. Not only did it take us away from the tiresome grind of reading text books and taking oral and written quizzes, but living out there afforded us delicious meals. The cook was famous for her homemade bread, rolls and pies and there was an unlimited amount of rich, whole milk, freshly-churned butter and country eggs; all part of the therapy for the patients. This, plus rest, was the only treatment for tuberculosis known at the time. Later pneumothorax (the collapsing of the affected lung with air) and chemotherapy would be used, the latter so successful that thirty years later, almost all the sanitaria were closed or turned over to other types of illnesses.

But this was 1930 and many patients were slowly dying of this *White Plague* with no hope of survival. They could be diagnosed from across the room with their flushed faces, emaciation and the characteristic, incongruously cheerful expressions. For some reason, the tuberculosis toxin seemed to stimulate them and to occur in such famous authors as Robert Louis Stevenson, Thomas Mann, D.H. Lawrence and Katherine Mansfield.

Students made rounds early every morning with Dr. James Murphy, the handsome, white-haired, medical director of the sanitarium. He knew each patient personally and made the examinations particularly interesting because he gave a good history of each one. He was sensitive and sympathetic, waiting until we left each bedside before giving a prognosis, which, in most cases, was particularly bleak. He insisted every student wash their hands thoroughly after each examination because these were "open cases" with live tuberculosis organisms on the patients' skin and lips. They were, essentially, very infectious.

Each student was assigned a patient as though they were seeing the patient for the first time, taking the history, ordering laboratory work and examining on their own. Then when the Section came to this patient on rounds, the students had to present the case and answer any questions about it. This was quite educational, since it was the pattern of *making rounds* that we would follow all during internship and residency.

I loved every minute of it.   This was what practicing medicine was all about, seeing patients, working them up; and making the diagnosis, prognosis and treatment. The only sad part was that there was so little hope for most of these cases.

My patient was Mary, a pretty girl of about sixteen with long brown hair and a trusting smile.

"Have you any idea how you contracted this disease?" I asked.

"No, there is no one among my friends or family who has it. I do have a grandfather who coughs a lot. *Chronic bronchitis,* they say it is, but he never has been examined."

"Never had an X-ray or sputum test?"

"No. But he has to come to the clinic tomorrow."

It was a common story. Many old people were carriers with long standing infections, dangerous to others but not to themselves.

Fortunately, all relatives and close contacts of the patients had to report to the sanitarium's outpatient clinic and many new cases were discovered in this way. It was called *case finding.* They were isolated until their sputum was negative, if ever.

It was while I was examining my patient that Ernie appeared.

He was a classmate who lived in the sanitarium, working as an intern, earning money to put himself through medical school. I'd never paid much attention to him because he was in another section, except to notice his striking resemblance to Humphrey Bogart. He was not handsome, but had a certain dynamic flair.

"What are you doing, playing doctor?" he asked.

I flushed. I still minded being teased about my chosen profession.

"This is a most interesting patient. Very little physical findings but a hectic type of temperature and many Koch's bacilli in the sputum."

"Great! I'm looking for organisms in my dog experiments." He sounded most enthusiastic.

I wanted to know what kind of research he was doing, so he invited me to come to his laboratory that evening and he would show me.

I had a hard time finding the lab. It was in the back of the morgue, a dismal, one-story, white frame building with Ernie's bedroom next to the dog lab. It smelled of animals, antiseptic and the decay of dead bodies.

Ernie was waiting for me with an eager expression on his *Bogie* face. We took a tour through the quiet morgue. Only two long, lean, still shapes lay under white sheets.

"Not much business today," said Ernie with his toothy smile.

I shuddered. Imagine living in a morgue! "Don't you mind having your room here?"

"Why should I? Nobody snores and I have my board and room free with very few duties except moving a body off the ward once in a while. Besides, I get to do research with Dr. Murphy, who is one swell guy."

"What kind of research?"

"I'll show you," he said, guiding me into a small room with four dog cages in it. There were only two occupants of the cages and they greeted Ernie enthusiastically, barking happily and wagging their tails.

"What do you do with those poor things?" My love for animals showed.

He laughed. "Nothing so terrible. Maybe you can be my assistant and help me sometime. There has never been a primary complex established in a dog. That is made by implanting live tubercle bacilli in the lung and watching the lesion grow by following it with a series of X-rays. If we could do this, it would be a scientific triumph."

"How do you get the bacteria into the lung?"

"I blow them in through a tube while the dog is anesthetized."

I was shocked. "Isn't that terribly dangerous for you? What if the dog coughed and you inhaled the living organisms? Wouldn't you get T.B?"

He smiled a grim smile.   "That's the breaks.   What bacteriological research doesn't have its hazards?"

All at once I felt a surge of admiration for this strangely appealing person who was pioneering in an unexplored area.

"I'd love to help. When can we start?"

"Atta girl! We'll begin next week."

The dog was a toy collie, a pet of Ernie's. He was about six years old, gentle and loyal. He particularly enjoyed the walks Ernie took him on twice daily through the walled in grounds where he could romp freely.

I went with them whenever I did not have duties on the ward and had fun throwing a ball and watching Walter retrieve it.

Ernie said he had never known a girl he could have such a good time with and I blossomed under his frank admiration.

Finally the day came when we had to inject the tubercle bacilli through Walter's throat. It was a gloomy, wet Sunday so the walk was cut short, then we returned to the lab and we put Walter on the examining table. He wagged his tail because he thought it was some kind of a game. I put my arms around him.

"Now don't get all choked up," said Ernie. "He won't feel a thing." And he skillfully injected an anesthetic into a vein which showed clearly above Walter's right paw. The dog promptly curled up and went to sleep.

"Here is where you come in," Ernie said. "Hold his mouth open while I insert this plastic tube in his trachea. Don't let him move!"

I grasped the dog's head firmly and pulled his jaws open. With a tongue blade holding Walter's tongue down, Ernie quickly threaded a narrow plastic tube past the dog's epiglottis into the trachea and on into the right main bronchus which we checked with the fluoroscope.

"I'm putting it down as far as it will go," said Ernie, "because we want to place the tubercle bacilli in the smallest bronchial possible."

I watched his deft movements with admiration. Walter was still sleeping peacefully.

"Now for the blow tube." Ernie reached over to the sterile table and took the prepared glass tubing which contained a suspension of the lethal bacteria.

I held my breath as he put one end into his mouth and carefully blew three long breaths through it.

"Well," said Ernie, "that's that."

I was relieved when the procedure was over and Walter was replaced in his cage. I did not know whether or not I hoped the experiment would be a success. For Ernie's and Dr. Murphy's sakes I hoped the primary complex would develop and they would publish the results in a prominent medical journal. On the other hand, for Walter's sake I hoped the germs would not grow because the poor dog might die of tuberculosis. I guessed I was too sentimental, but I could not help it.

Ernie was elated, talking excitedly all through dinner. After dinner Ernie and I went back to his spare, clean room, lounged on his cot and listened to his collection of classical records — early Bartok, Mahler and Schumann.

I was sorry when the two week's clerkship was over and I had to go back to the daily grind of watching operations in the surgical amphitheater. I wondered whether I would ever see Ernie again, but I did not have to wait long because in the next large lecture, he sat down beside me, much to Kenny's disgust.

"How's my research partner?"

I laughed, "I still have nightmares about poor Walter. How is he?"

"Oh, full of spit and vinegar, as usual. But he misses you. How would you like to take a walk with him next Sunday?"

Although I had a surgery quiz on Monday, I agreed eagerly. There was something about Ernie which made me feel needed and I liked this feeling.

All my life, I had been taken care of by my parents. Whenever I wanted to help around the house, Mother had told me to go practice the piano or do my lessons or, if I had nothing to do, to go sit in the sun. And since I hated household chores (who didn't?) I escaped willingly. But, as a result, I never felt I was contributing anything and now I did. Maybe Walter and Ernie did need me. I would find out.

So the small, clean room in the morgue with the dog cages next door and the bodies down the hall became a haven for the two of us and our friendship deepened. The other students watched the twosome develop. They whispered and shook their heads knowingly.

One evening when I was entranced by Debussy's La Mer. Ernie took me in his arms and kissed me long and searchingly. I pulled away and looked at him in surprise.

"I wanted to see whether a kiss could bring out the same dreamy expression in your eyes that Debussy did."

I laughed, "Well, did it?"

"Not quite, but I have hopes. Maybe with practice I can produce it." And he tried again.

It became a lighthearted romance with much laughter, interspersed with serious discussions of medical topics and philosophy, frequent subjects of medical students.

It would last until I completed medical school.

ENDINGS AND BEGINNINGS

Cook County Hospital was a large, tan stone building occupying an entire block on the West Side of Chicago. Its capacity of over two thousand patient beds was, in the early nineteen thirties, the largest hospital in the world. As a result of this and a superior attending staff, the teaching potential of the institution was excellent. Cook County received so many applications for internship that examinations were given to senior medical students from all over the United States.

I had taken a course to prepare for the exam and had written it during four trying hours in February of my senior year.

When the day came for the posting of the lucky winners, the Senior Class gathered anxiously about the bulletin board in the medical school. The three months waiting had been filled with anxiety because if each student failed to pass the examination, he or she would have to find another internship. Many had written to other institutions, but had held off accepting other offers in the hope of *making County* – the dream of their life.

The trouble with waiting was that the positions at other hospitals were filling up fast and the student might end up with no place to intern or, at least, an internship in a small hospital with an inferior staff.

Barbara was at my side, as usual, providing moral support. She and her fiancé, Ty, had accepted internships at University of Illinois Research Hospital, a good teaching institution, so she was not involved.

I turned to her. "Won't they ever come, I can't stand much more of this waiting?"

Barbara said, "Don't worry you'll make it. You made Phi Beta Kappa and Alpha Omega Alpha, so there's no doubt about this."

I shook my head. "I didn't know the mechanism of breech delivery. Maybe that will keep me out."

We were interrupted by a great shout from our classmates as the little dean came bustling importantly around the corner of the corridor with the results in his hand.

"Now, now! Don't be so impatient." he admonished the crowd. "Let me through. Let me through." He shouldered his way to the bulletin board and firmly attached the list with four thumb tacks.

There was a great surge forward and the dean could barely escape.

Howls came from many delighted students.

"I made it. I made it!" shouted Leon, the one with an Egyptian appearance. He turned to me while I stood on tip toes trying to see over the tall men.

"And you made it too," he smiled at me, "Eighteenth place."

Eighteenth out of one hundred. Well, it was better than nothing. Although it did not give me much choice of service. Mixed emotions filled my eyes with tears.

Barbara hugged me, "I am so glad for you! I knew you could do it. Let's go have a Coke to celebrate."

My next thought was to inform Father. I left Barbara and hurried to his office.

He looked up from his writing and smiled. "Well, Dorothy? I can see you've got some good news to tell me. Is that right?"

I laughed, "Pretty good, I made County but only eighteenth place."

"That's fine. You shouldn't complain about that," he said. "I'm proud of you. County's a fine institution, although a little large."

I knew he said that because he had wanted me to go into research instead of practicing. He was a scientist through and through.

I told him, "There are lab people like you and there are other people like me. I like taking care of patients instead of looking at test tubes!"

He gave up without a struggle, knowing I was right for once.

So the fourth year came to an end with two main events coming up. The first, of course, was graduation.

My father was dressed in his regal robes with Columbia University's Ph.D. blue and gold hood draped over the shoulders and back. He looked most dignified, even though his mortar board was tilted at a slightly rakish angle. He was the Grand Marshall of the procession so he had to get there early. My plain black robe looked drab by comparison, but I did not mind because it meant the end of four trying years.

The auditorium of the local theater was rapidly filling up with spectators, relatives and friends of the graduates.

In the main section were scattered couples here and there. Most of them lower middle-class persons dressed in their Sunday best. Many of them had sacrificed economically to put their sons through medical school. Nanny, Aunt Alice and Mother were seated in the section reserved for faculty family.

I waved to them and left to join the milling group of second year students waiting to line up for their BS degree and fourth year students happily waiting to become MD's – Doctors of Medicine. A long sought after goal finally achieved. What a happy day! They were noisy and animated.

I looked around and saw my friends. Barbara with her ever-present Ty; Kenny, insouciant, sardonic as ever; the Egyptian-looking Leon surrounded by his admiring clique; and Ernie staring at me with his prominent brown eyes as though he could devour me in a single glance. Soon, they would all go their separate ways to various internships scattered across the country. I felt sad at the thought.

My father was lining them up in alphabetical order, so that each diploma would get to the right student. I heard one of them say, "Old Doc Welker looks as hard boiled as ever!"

The strains of Pomp and Circumstance, played by a small local orchestra, floated out of the orchestra pit. The seniors of the class of 1931 marched in. I settled my mortar board more securely and gave Barbara's hand a reassuring squeeze. How often I had done that in the past, before exams especially. When we reached our seats the faculty marched in with the least important first.

I recognized many of them. The Histology instructor, Isador Press, with his frog face; the ambidextrous Anatomy professor, Dr. Kitchner; Dr. Darcy, the head of Physiology; Dr. Landau, the E.N.T. Department Head, teller of the off color jokes; Dr. Seed of surgery who gave all the girls C's; Dr. Watson, Dean of the Professional school; and President Kinley, the head of Urbana – Champaign and Chicago campuses.

I thought of the quotation from the Bible, "And the least shall be first," only, in this case, "the great shall be last," and Father was shepherding all of them in! I really was proud of him.

When we were arranged, the President introduced a clergyman who gave a short invocation and we were seated.

I thought the talk by a visiting scientist would never end. Then came the presenting of the diplomas by the President and the Dean.

My hand was much colder than the Dean's when he shook it and I descended the steps with relief.

Getting my Master of Science diploma came next, but by then I was numb and did not mind it. All these years of work ending with a handshake and two pieces of parchment.

The announcing of the members of Alpha Omega Alpha Medical Society honoring twelve members of our class came next and I had to go back up those same stairs once more because I was tied for third place in the class with Ernest Otto van der Aue, my OB partner. As I passed Dr. Seed, I could not help giving him a triumphant nod. That misogynist!

The next big event was Barbara and Ty's wedding. It was scheduled for the day after graduation.

I was asked to be the maid of honor. Mother and I had been working for weeks on a pink, dotted Swiss dress with a huge full skirt, a tiny waist and one hundred yards of narrow, Valenciennes lace. My mother teased me, saying I should have been the bride. She had found a wide brimmed, Leghorn, straw hat with long, pink streamers on it. When I was all dressed I felt more glamorous than I ever had in my life.

One of Barbara's friends was a florist and supplied free flowers for the church and Barbara's and my huge bouquets. Barbara's had white orchids and gardenias and mine was a closely packed combination of yellow daisies, blue bachelor buttons, small white asters and tiny pink rose buds. It was over fourteen inches in diameter and must have had more than a 100 blooms in it.

I had to walk alone down a long aisle in the large Catholic church. It seemed endless and, although we had practiced it over and over the evening before, I was shaking so much that many of the flowers fell out of my bouquet.

The bride's family and friends, mostly Bohemians, sat on the right side of the church and on the left sat Ty's Polish family and friends. It was quite a contrast because, at that time, Bohemians and Poles were not too fond of each other.

I looked ahead and saw Ty and his best man, Fred, standing tall and handsome by the right side of the altar. Fred was a classmate of mine in medical school who I knew only slightly. Finally, I reached the altar and turned sideways so I could see the tiny flower girl and little ring bearer approaching us proudly.

Then came Barbara, rosy, very serious looking and lovelier than I'd ever seen her. Her satin lace dress had a long train and she wore a filmy veil covering her face and falling gracefully down her back. She had a little circle of lilies-of-the-valley as a crown.

Her handsome father led her to the altar and the ceremony began.

I didn't understand the words, which were Latin. My job was to straighten Barbara's train as she changed from place to place at the altar, kneeling at various locations. Finally, after presenting her bouquet to the statue of the Virgin Mary, the bride joined the groom for a kiss and the happy final procession out of the church.

Ernie, who was waiting to go to the reception with me, said, "Well, if that ceremony does not tie them up for good, nothing will!"

The wedding dinner was fun with much drinking of toasts and teasing of the handsome young couple. After it was over, everyone left in a romantic mood. For some time Ernie had been asking me to marry him and, finally, I consented.

Still under the influence of Barbara and Ty's charming wedding, we drove down to the City Hall the next day and waited in line for our license. There were several nondescript couples ahead of us. Among them, one older man with a young bride and two teenagers. I became more nervous as time went on.

I looked at Ernie and asked myself, Do you want to spend the rest of your life with this man? The answer was a tentative, "Yes." Then I asked myself, "Would you like to have him be the father of your children?" and the answer was a definite, "No."

The thing that made me doubtful about marrying Ernie was the fact that he liked to drink. To me, who had been raised in a strict Pennsylvania Dutch household where heavy liquor, or even beer, was not allowed, seeing Ernie have three cocktails or more was not appealing.

I had mentioned this to him before and he'd answered seriously, "As long as you are not used to it, I will give it up.

When I found out that his alcoholic father had committed suicide, I began to wonder whether the promises he made so glibly now would be broken after marriage. All of this went through my head as we stood waiting in line, so then and there I made one of the most important decisions of my life.

"Oh Ernie," I said, "I'm so sorry, but I can not go through with this. Let's get out of here."

He was amazed and angry, but did not try to dissuade me. He knew it would be of no use.

We went back to my Oak Park home and told my parents. After Ernie left, my mother said, "I am so glad you decided on your own not to marry Ernie. Your father and I did not feel you were making a wise choice, but we knew if we tried to talk you out of it, you probably would turn to him all the more, so we kept out of it."

I said, "It must have been hard to do."

Mother smiled her little secret smile and said, "It was."

Later, Ernie told me, "I hated giving you up, but it was worse to give up your parents!" This reinforced the feeling I had made the right decision.

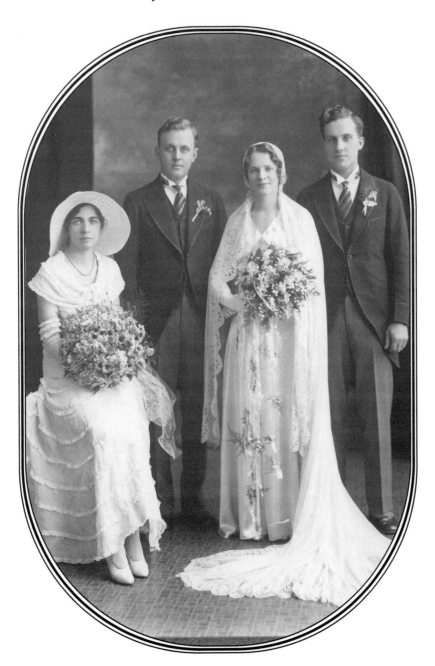

Barbara's Wedding

A LITTLE CHUTZPA

After a few delightful weeks with my parents at the family cottage in Northern Wisconsin, I returned to Chicago by train to start my internship.

My father and mother had driven me to the Minong Station and, as the train pulled out, I felt a bit wistful at seeing the two of them standing alone on the little country platform. They were both dressed in their khaki fishing outfits: huge boots, suede jackets, jodhpurs and fishing hats. I thought my mother looked a little sad.

After all, this was a large fork in the road. I was embarking on a career and leaving them further and further behind.

I sighed and thought, "Dorothy, you are a sentimental fool! You've worked eight years for this moment and now you are regretting leaving your folks!" I turned my thoughts to the excitement of being an intern. What services would I get and who would be my senior?

Internship in those days was eighteen months long. I would be a junior intern for six months, a middler for six months and a senior intern for six months.

The big advantage for a junior was being chosen by a good senior whose job it was to train the younger intern in the services which the senior had picked. Having written eighteenth place, I felt I wouldn't have much chance of getting a good senior.

The interns met in the Warden's quarters. That was the name

given to the Administrator of Cook County Hospital because he had been Warden of the County Jail for many years. I thought how appropriate that title was for the patients were all more or less prisoners in this vast institution of 2,000 beds.

Warden Jamison was a short, squat, balding man with deep creases in his face and a sudden unpredictable smile.

"Well," he said, "I see you all made it. Are you ready to chose your services? Pair off into numbers one and one here, two and two next and etc."

We did so. I was astounded by my senior. He looked like an ex-prize fighter with large shoulders, short neck, cauliflower ears and a broken nose. His name was Charlie Finklestein and he smiled at me warmly.

"I never thought I'd draw a woman junior," he said, "but I like it."

I nodded, speechless.

"I'm going into obstetrics and gynecology," he said. "I hope you'll be interested in that because it will be our first service."

"How do you know?" I asked.

He drew me to one side of the group and whispered confidentially, "I have a friend who wants to have the psychiatric service. That comes way down the list. So he will pick the best Gyne service and I'll pick Psych and we'll switch."

He looked at me for approval, but my expression was one of bewilderment. "Is that permitted?" I asked.

"Oh course it is, if we do it!" He grinned. I was to find out that was his motto and he always got away with it.

So we ended up with the Barette-Fishman Service which was the best in the Gyne department. All because Charlie's friend had written third place and wanted to be a psychiatrist and Charlie had *Chutzpah.*

Charlie Finklestein was one of the homeliest men I had ever seen. Some friend of his said, "Charlie has an identical twin brother. Would you believe it? Two guys who look like that?"

But once I got to know the inner part of him, the outer part didn't matter, in fact the contrast made him even more appealing, for he was kind, considerate and very Jewish. He taught me many Yiddish phrases such as "Obe Gesund" (as long as you're healthy) and "Kein-a-Hora" (no evil eye), which came in handy when I was taking histories from Jewish patients.

Every Friday night while I took his calls, Charlie went home to a good Jewish dinner and afterwards brought back a tray for me. I learned to like chicken soup with matzo balls, home made challe – twisted egg bread, gefilte fish, tzimmis – a sweet carrot dish, and helze – which was the skin of a chicken neck full of a delicious flour, egg and fat mixture. I also loved Mrs. Finklestein's delicious butter-küchen. What fun it was for me to eat this weekly banquet while perched on a stool in the Gyne Ward office and laughing at Charlie's jokes.

The Gyne Ward, or Ward 40 as it was called, was a dismal place in the old building, consisting of one long room with thirty beds lined up on each side of it. The *sun porch*, misnamed since it was not a porch and certainly had no sun, was a smaller room located off to one side. This was really a hell hole stuffed with cancer patients and filled with moans and the stench of decay. I dreaded making rounds in there since the patients were suffering so. Morphine was injected when *necessary* but that phrase was open to the interpretation of the head nurse who was constantly worried about addiction. With the prognoses so bad in most of the patients, I wondered what difference it made. They surely would not get shots in heaven.

Dr. Barette, the head of the Gyne Department, was a tall, handsome, white haired, husky surgeon who met with Charlie and me two evenings a week and decided whether or not the patients we had chosen were qualified for operations.

I had written the history of each one and had my examination checked by Charlie. He was anxious to become as good a surgeon as Dr. Barette, who was tops in his field.

Charlie wheeled each patient into a small examining room and I presented the case history followed by a discussion of the findings by Dr. Barette and Charlie.

Being a charity institution in a large city like Chicago, most of the patients in Gyne were poor, uneducated women. The frequent diagnosis was fibroids, tumors of the uterus which often bleed profusely. These women were naturally apprehensive about being operated upon and asked that their *pleasure* be left in. Charlie, who was very sympathetic, always assured them it would be.

"If they think we won't remove anything which interferes with their sex life," Charlie told me, "then they will be all right afterward."

"But do we have to take out their ovaries too, in all cases?" I asked.

"Sometimes yes and sometimes no, depending on whether they have cysts, other tumors or infection in them or in their tubes," Charlie answered. He was very pleased with his role as teacher and really spent a lot of time and energy instructing his eager young pupil. I was grateful for his information, especially after some of the sad experiences I had with instructors in medical school.

Dr. Barette was particularly pleasant, which was a surprise because he had a reputation of being somewhat austere and standoffish. In the operating room, his routine was always the same. He never *turned* any operation to the senior, which irked Charlie to no end. Resigned to the fact that he wouldn't get hands on experience, Charlie watched each move carefully, enjoying the two handed technique that Barette was noted for. Thankfully, the other doctor in the service was more willing to allow Charlie to operate so he got his experience that way.

Sometimes we had more complicated cases, such as disseminated cancer of the uterus, and had to do more extensive surgery than that of simply removing fibroids.

My hand's were deft and I liked sewing and cutting. It reminded me of dress making which Mother had taught me at home.

Sometimes Charlie got annoyed at not being given any "work" as he called it. So when Dr. Barette said, "You may close now, Doctor," Charlie would turn to me and say, "It's up to you, Doctor," and walk away.

That was my shining hour and I delightedly *closed*, that is, sewed up the patient's incision with the help of the surgical nurse.

At first, the nurses were antagonistic to this *hen-medic* in the Operating Room, but as time went on, they became much more accepting of me and some even tried to help me.

Dr. Barette took a liking to me and, one day, after standing and working all morning in a hot operating room (before the blessing of air conditioning), he took off his gloves, mask and gown and then said to me, "How about a few sets of tennis?"

I was ready to lie down and rest, but I couldn't admit it to this sixty-five year old giant so I said, "I'd love to if you don't mind a rank amateur."

Barette laughed loudly and said, "Anyone who played on the team in Urbana - Champaign could hardly be called a rank amateur."

So we played several sets of tennis which went fast because Dr. Barette was an expert and could go from the back line to the net in three or four giant strides. Besides that, he played with both hands, switching the racket with lightening speed. The scores were usually 6-0, 6-1 or 6-2, with "guess who" as victor?

Toward the end of the three months Gyne service, Barette allowed me to perform a vaginal hysterectomy much to my delight and terror. Of course he was there to assist me and Charlie stood by too, but with a disappointed expression on his face.

By this time, I had just about decided I would be an obstetrical and gynecological specialist because operating came so easy to me. However, merely doing the operation was one thing, taking good postoperative care was another, as I would find out only too soon.

The operation went very well with me remembering step by step Dr. Barette's excellent technique. I gave a great sigh of relief when it was over and was thrilled when Dr. Barette said, "That was well done, Doctor Dorothy. I believe you have the makings of a good surgeon."

My elation soon turned to anxiety. I felt so responsible for this patient, a fifty year old, pleasant little woman, that I sat up with her all night. I checked her vital signs and worried when she gave little moans of pain. By morning I did not know which of us felt worse.

Charlie came around early to make rounds and found me half asleep in a chair by the patient's bed. "What in hell are you doing here?" he asked. "You look as though you've been up all night."

"I have," I admitted sheepishly. "I couldn't sleep so I came over and stayed here."

Charlie snorted, "A fine surgeon you'll make – killing yourself with worry over each patient! What would you do if a patient that you had operated on really went bad?" I knew he was still annoyed that Dr. Barette had *turned* an operation to me – a junior, instead of to him – a lofty senior.

Those were the days of very few residents, when interns got to do as many operations as residents did in later years. And, at a big charity institution, that was quite a few. In spite of that, the risk to the patient was minimal with the attending surgeon monitoring the whole operation.

However, after a few experiences of this kind, with me worried all night about my patients, I discovered there was much more to surgery than having a good pair of hands. I decided that I would go into some less emotion-laden profession such as Dermatology, Radiology or Pediatrics. I would have to see which service I preferred.

INTERN DISCOVERS KNIFE

The next service was Male Medicine. This was a seventy bed ward in a clean new building and in some ways a lot more pleasant than Gyne.

However, the first night I was on call made me wonder about how great it was going to be.

There were five female interns, including myself, in the dormitory building. I was just drifting off to sleep in my room, shared with two of the other female interns, when the phone rang.

"Dr. Welker?" an anxious nurse was calling. "Please come over to your ward immediately. One of the patients has hung himself."

I put on my white uniform and ran about a block between the buildings. On the way over I kept thinking about how to treat the man if he were still alive. I had never seen a hanging. I shivered from cold and fear.

The intern had wheeled Mr. Polacheck's bed into the *dying room* which was what the patients called the tiny cubicle just off the nurses' station.

I was horrified by the sight of this man's purple face, bulging eyes and protuberant tongue. I felt his pulse. It was still palpable but weak and thready. The marks of a rope made a narrow bruise about his neck.

This nurse had started one unit of 5% dextrose intravenously to combat shock. She asked me, "Now what?"

I wished I knew. I felt completely helpless. Where was Charlie? I called his room but found he had signed out to me.

I was very grateful Mrs. Smith-Jones was substituting for the regular night nurse on Ward 26. I had seen this experienced nurse work before and I respected her knowledge and aptitude. I knew she asked that question to see whether I had treated such a case before. I decided I would not try to bluff this dedicated woman. I felt she knew more about emergency care than many interns did.

"Really, Mrs. Smith-Jones," I said, looking straight into her wise eyes. "I'm sure you know a lot more about treating such a case than I do. So I'll ask you, what next?"

She smiled and from then on we were friends.

I wanted to get an X-ray of the man's cervical spine but I was afraid to move him and no portable X-rays could be taken at that hour of the night. We decided to fashion a make shift collar with a large firm bath towel and run a rope on each side of it over the top of the bedstead with ten-lb. weights at each end.

The nurse and I secured the unconscious man's feet to the foot of the bed and then waited, after starting three liters of oxygen by a plastic tube in his nose. Slowly, slowly his color improved. His tongue became nearly its normal size and his pulse was stronger. He was going to make it.

Mrs. Smith-Jones helped me with information for charting the patient. The man had been admitted to the ward because he'd attempted suicide that afternoon at home. He'd had an argument with his seventeen year old son about the son's taking dope and was discouraged at his son's negative response. The policeman on the case brought him to the hospital to be watched, but the man brought some rope with him and when the attendants were off the ward he hung himself in the bathroom.

Fortunately, Mrs. Smith-Jones cut him down in time.

I stayed with him through the night and, in the morning, turned him over to the suicide counselor.

Another interesting case that came my way was that of Hans Anderson, a burly, doltish-looking Swede who had seen better days. He had descended the economic ladder and finally landed at the bottom, belonging to a group of tramps who lived in hobo jungles beside railroad tracks.

He was admitted to Ward 26 for diagnosis and treatment of convulsions of unknown origin. He told me he'd been suffering from these mysterious seizures for about seven years.

I couldn't get much more of a history out of him because his memory was blurry, with no accurate recollection of dates and places. He knew he'd been in several hospitals but had no idea of what the doctors had said.

I found nothing on a complete physical examination except an enlarged liver and vague neurological signs. His brain waves showed a slight abnormality in the left frontal region. So I, being meticulous as usual, ordered anterior, posterior and lateral views of the skull.

The next day the Head of Radiology asked me to come right over to the X-ray department. I went over wondering what they found.

"How long have you had this patient?" Dr. Henderson asked excitedly.

"He just came in two days ago." I answered.

"What did he come in for?"

"Convulsions of seven years' duration."

"My God, where has he been all this time?"

"In and out of various hospitals without any help."

Dr. Henderson gave a scornful shout. "I should think not! Take a look at this!" He showed me the skull films.

I gasped. There was a four inch knife blade imbedded in the left frontal lobe of the brain.

"The poor man! No wonder he has convulsions." I shook my head. "Why has no one ever taken an X-ray before?"

I hurried back to the ward and found Hans sitting up in bed staring dully ahead of him.

"When can I get out of here?" he asked.

"Not for a while I'm afraid. Let's go over your history again. Were you ever in any fights?"

"Ya, lots of them, especially when we boys got to drinking."

"Did any of the men fight with knives?"

"My friend Johanson cut me once on my head and I fell in the fire. The boys dragged me out and took me to a hospital."

"Where?"

"I don't remember . . . somewhere . . . maybe Denver. It was seven or eight years ago."

"Did you have convulsions before that?"

"No, I don't think so. After, I guess."

I couldn't wait to show the films to Charlie. For once his attention was diverted from Gyne. He told a friend about it who worked for the Chicago Tribune and soon, I was besieged by reporters. It was front page Associated Press copy complete with an awful picture of me pointing to Hans forehead and another picture of the knife showing plainly on X-ray. The headlines read, INTERN FINDS KNIFE IN BRAIN.

Soon the phone was ringing with friends from all over the United States calling me up to congratulate me. One telephone call was from the Medical Administrator of the hospital, the dreaded Dr. Mark Meyer. He was an autocrat and everyone trembled at his summons, and he wanted to see me.

I was not at all afraid. In fact I was happy to be recognized by the great man. I stood in front of his desk with a pleased smile on my face. He kept on working for several minutes and then said gruffly without looking up, "Sit down, why are you just standing there?"

This was hardly a congratulation. I sat obediently. More waiting. Finally he gave me a sidelong glance.

"I hear you are becoming quite famous."

"Not really," I said

He glared at me.

"Have you ever heard of our regulations concerning press

releases?"

I shook my head.

"Didn't the Warden warn you about talking to reporters without sending them to me first?"

Suddenly it dawned on me. The man was jealous of my notoriety. I usurped his authority.

"What do you have to say for yourself? Do you know I can have your internship canceled for such an offense?"

I bit my lower lip to keep from blurting out, "You old fool! Being envious of a twenty-six year-old intern!" My silence irritated him.

"Answer me! Don't just sit there!"

"I'm sorry, Dr. Meyer, but I didn't know I was supposed to report this case to you."

He looked slightly mollified.

"Well, as long as you understand that in the future nothing goes to the media without my consent, I will let you off this time."

I felt that bowing down and kissing his ring was expected, but instead backed out quietly. "What an ass!" I thought.

Fortunately for Hans Anderson, the knife was successfully removed from his brain and all convulsions ceased.

Male medicine was a mixture of all kinds of chronic heart disease with decompensation. Several kinds of inoperable cancers had ascites, an accumulation of fluid in the abdomen. I felt very sorry whenever a new patient was admitted with a huge abdomen filled with fluid, because it meant draining it. This was the accepted method in those days.

Charlie showed me how to do it. We scrubbed the patient's abdomen, thoroughly painted it with tincture of iodine from his umbilicus down to his pubis and anesthetized the skin, muscles and the peritoneum. Then we inserted a trochar, a hideous looking instrument with sharp edges and a hollow inside. After it had been inserted, with hopes we would not puncture any intestines, we pulled out the inside stylette and clear yellow fluid gushed forth. Sometimes there was as much as a gallon and once it was released the patient felt better.

However it often filled up again so the process had to be repeated frequently. That was my task and I dreaded it. When the fluid accumulated rapidly we inserted a tube and had it run out by gravity. The problem was it often became infected and this was a serious complication.

Another task I despised had to do with the Halsted Street bums who drank anything they could lay their hands on – often wood alcohol. It was extremely poisonous to the system sometimes causing blindness, so the tramps' stomachs had to be washed out as soon as possible.

I had to insert a large tube in their stomachs, through the nose and down the throat, and pump out the disgusting smelling stuff. The smell of wood alcohol still takes me back to those unpleasant hours in male medicine.

The only comic relief was furnished by Mike, a huge, muscular man, who offered his services one day. After a particularly unpleasant half hour with a struggling, filthy, swearing, old reprobate, he appeared in the doorway of the examining room and said, "Say listen, Doc. How would you like a hand?"

I liked this man. He was more or less a permanent resident in the ward. He had been manager of the animal train for Barnum & Bailey's Circus and really knew how to handle men and other animals.

He suffered from a bleeding peptic ulcer on which he refused to have surgery. After three or four weeks in the ward, he would go out with the condition *arrested*, but not for long. His comrades welcomed him back with a big party and, because he could not resist the drinks, he always landed back on Ward 26 again, bleeding as before.

I accepted his help gladly and after a few pungent words and strong physical restraint, the patient cooperated. This then became routine and the patients passed the word around that the woman doctor had a helper that was not to be tampered with. All Mike had to do was stand in the doorway with his arms folded and the swearing and struggling stopped. Life became a lot easier for me after that.

Another person who was more or less a fixture in the ward was a handsome American Indian in his early twenties. Since the junior resident had to run urine tests each day, I trained him to do the simple dip test and readings of specific gravity. He was eager to learn and became quite accurate in performing everything but the microscopic examinations.

This saved me a great deal of time. I was inundated with all the history taking, examinations and rounds of the ward, because Charlie was not interested in Male Medicine at all. He had his goal firmly in mind, to be the best Gyne surgeon in the United States, so he spent very little time in the ward. As a result, I had an enormous load on my shoulders. I was working eighteen to twenty hours a day and was often too tired to eat. My one Friday evening banquet was my only balanced meal of the week.

Charlie, kind as he was, had a blind spot for anything that kept him out of the operating room. He did not realize that I was getting thinner and more tired day by day. I called Charlie up one evening.

"Do you mind watching the ward tonight?" I asked. "I am going to spend the night with Barbara over at Illinois Research Hospital. I need a break."

He agreed.

Ty was away for the night so Barbara and I had a great girl to girl chat. After going to bed I tossed about restlessly thinking of all the things we'd discussed. Suddenly, I had a severe coughing spell and could not stop. I felt a rush of sputum in the back of my throat and a salty taste in my mouth.

Barbara turned on the light and gasped as she saw a stream of blood on my sheet.

"What shall I do?" Barbara asked me.

"Call Charlie," was all I could say.

He came over immediately. He took one look at me and said, "Oh my God!"

He picked me up, all eighty-five pounds of me, and carried me the one block between Barbara's and the Cook County Hospital infirmary.

Since I didn't want to bother the attending man on call, the nurse put me to bed and Charlie settled down, sitting on the corridor floor with his back against my door. It was a long night.

The next day there was a serious consultation with my father, our family physician, Dr. Chauvet, and the radiologist. Although there was nothing specific on the X-rays of my chest, the fact that I had lost so much weight and was so exhausted made it mandatory for me to drop out of my internship for quite a while.

Father took me and my belongings home. I rebelled furiously, but it did no good. What Dr. William Henry Welker said was law. And a good thing I listened, too, because it possibly saved my life.

Years later, a large calcified lymph node showed up in the hilus of my lung, probably the result of exposure to the live tubercle bacilli in Ernie's experiments. Both the collie, Walter, and I had been inoculated and had developed a primary complex − a successful ending to the experiment, but not a happy ending of my first two years' service as a junior intern.

LOVE AT LONE LARCH

After spending nine months at home in Oak Park, being colossally bored, I was very happy to arrive at the Lone Larch Cottage, Father's name for the lodge he had built on a three mile-long lake in Northern Wisconsin.

I lay prone and completely relaxed on the narrow pier. The hot sun warmed my shoulders and the wide boards felt firm beneath me. With one arm acting as a pillow, I reached over the edge of the pier and touched the cool water with the fingers of the other hand. To be relaxed and comfortable in all one's relationships, to be certain of one's friends, their loyalty and strength, never to doubt or wonder. I daydreamed blissfully of a friendly utopia in the perfect setting of the Northwoods.

Dark green trees marched triumphantly down to the water's edge, tier after tier from the highest hilltop down the descending steps of strings in the third movement of Beethoven's Fifth Symphony. From the violins through the violas, cellos and straight down through the basses. Great symphonies and virgin forests have much in common; depth, mystery and startling beauty.

Occasionally, a white birch stood out against the dark green of the tamaracks like the stark motif of a flute; the flash of bright wings from leafy cover exploded like a brilliant scale of piccolos; the thumping of pheasants resounded like the pianissimo beat of the kettle drums. What joy to be a composer and put love of the woods into music — to capture the forest into interesting sound so clear and mystic that even the city-imprisoned ones could escape into arboreal vastness and breathe again and be refreshed.

I turned over to see the sky above, infinitely blue and tranquil. A deep sense of peace. Green treetops against translucent light and an answering exultation of the heart.

The pier trembled slightly as someone approached it from the shore. Grateful for this advance warning, I pulled myself back from my imaginary far places to the present world. Mother appeared at the boat house door loaded with fishing gear.

"Hurry up and get the oars," she called gaily. "Let's catch some supper."

I lazily pulled myself to a sitting position and then to my knees. From this vantage point mother appeared to me as she had in my childhood. Tall and lovely, her face flushed with enthusiasm and her eyes shining.

"I think you would rather fish than eat," I remarked.

"Well one thing's certain" said Mother, "if we don't fish, we don't eat."

Following the shore line in the light steel boat, I rowed carefully outside the drop-off so that we could cast over this sudden under water slope where the fish lay. We were happily silent, alert to the first suggestion of a follow or a strike, watching for the sudden swirls which were suggestive of a near miss. Tiny wavelets sparkled brilliantly in the sunlight and made little slapping sounds on the side of the boat.

"Fine time to be fishing — in the middle of the day!" I said looking at Mother perched on the edge of the stern seat, her right leg tucked under her. "You look as though a good sized walleye would pull you right into the lake."

At each cast she seemed to hover half over the lake and then she would return to her former position.

"Rotten form," she would say, laughing, "but it goes farther."

Mother liked the Northwoods, but in a different way from

my deep attachment to it. When Mother returned to our suburban home each year, she thought of Lone Larch occasionally with a pleasant nod of recognition. But I lived at Lake Gilmore and merely existed in other places. I felt a metamorphosis within myself the moment I stepped off the train at the little wooden station that reminded me of the toy depots one found under Christmas trees.

Each year when I arrived, it seemed as though all the sordidness and the competition of the city fell from me and I became light and free once more. The wind had a winey tang and I took long complete breaths. Even the tired, dusty, main street of Minong had a magical appeal, for it was the entry to the Northwoods. Mother had a saying, "Life begins at Lake Gilmore for Dorothy." It was true.

The fishing was poor that day and we came home sheepishly bearing one medium-sized bass. We were greeted by Father's skepticism as he waited on the boathouse steps. In his warm outdoor clothes, he bore no resemblance to the dignified professor of the other ten months of the year. In school, he was stern, severe and perfectly correct in an Oxford gray suit, white shirt, and authoritative, stiff-winged collar and a small black bow tie. Here at Lone Larch, he could be himself. The sight of him with his fishing hat pushed back, his pipe poking from his mouth at a jaunty angle and his face and hands a deep tan made me smile. Even the curling, gray hair on the back of his hands seemed to spring up sturdily with the sheer joy of living in the outdoors. His keen blue eyes took in the size of the fish.

"Cradle snatching again," he remarked dryly. "And at your age, too!"

We defied him by swinging the fish proudly as we walked up the steep steps to the cabin.

The sixty foot climb was long and tiring but it never seemed difficult to me for there were wild roses peeping out between each step, and wood lilies scattered here and there over the slope like stars fallen onto the green tangle.

The cabin, with is weathered logs, wide verandah and casement windows with tiny panes was a cool, friendly home. I stretched out on the porch swing and fell asleep. When I awoke an hour later, my first feeling was vague sense of pleasure, as though I were being gently stroked.

I tried to place the cause of this sensation and realized it came from a voice, pleasant and soothing that seemed to say, "All is well, don't worry. Nothing can hurt you. All is well," although the actual words were quite inaudible. I closed my eyes again, afraid to break the spell.

Why was it so few people and their voices seemed to match? Either the voice was like velvet and the individual's personality was like rough tweed or visa-versa.

Would this person, whoever he was, talking to my father measure up to his voice – so varied melodious and reassuring? I did not want to see him. I turned over and pretended to be asleep so I could keep the sound of that voice intact.

A few days later, the family drove to town for our weekly supply of groceries. The quarter mile private road which led from the front of the cabin to County Trunk I was narrow and winding, crisscrossed by globular and linear purplish shadows which stood out clearly against the yellow sand. The trees hung protectively about the road as though to hide it from a stranger's eye and clumps of blueberry bushes appeared on each side.

We drove past the mail box, symbol of Lone Larch's one tie to the township of Minong and onto the black-top road. This was more civilized with a bedraggled farm house every mile or so.

The first part of the six mile trip was delightful. It curved between large trees with an occasional glimpse of the lake through the dense foliage.

Halfway to town was a small waterfall where a stream entered another lake. There were several children fishing in a pond. Tattered little boys with patches on their overalls, looking like the colored pictures on the calendars of the 1890's. It was one of the changeless fundamentals, the relationship of a boy to his fishing pole.

"How's fishing?" I called and one of the boys answered by waving a string of tiny pumpkin seed fish in the air.

A few miles later we drove down the deserted main street of the town with three hundred inhabitants. Minong always seemed to me to be holding its breath, waiting for something that never happened.

My parents went into the local store while I sat outside wondering what it must be like to live in such a quiet village, without the hustle and bustle of a big city.

A young man passed, his high boots clumping rhythmically on the sidewalk. He had a gallant swing to his walk, lithe and free, which matched the cocky tilt of an old felt hat pulled down hard above one eye.

I wondered what he did for a living, for he had none of the discouraged stoop which labeled so many of the local men as sand farmers. He could not be a summer visitor; for they appeared obviously at odds with the scenery. He must be a native, I concluded, and went back to impatiently waiting for the return of my parents. They finally came out laden with bundles.

We stopped at a gas station and, while my parents were talking to the owner, the stranger approached the car from the other side and looked in at me. Mother and Father, being busy, did not notice him and there was nothing but this quiet look which passed between the two of us. Suddenly a new, wordless communication developed. I received the message of wondering admiration in his eyes and I knew he felt my completely unguarded surprise.

"Hello, Bill." my father said, getting in the drivers seat.

"Hello, Dr. Welker," he answered quietly.

He was the one. Bill's was the caressing voice I'd heard in my waking dream.

*   *   *   *   *

A week later, I decided to try my luck at catching a fish or two for supper again. I lay back lazily in the bottom of the row boat, my head resting against the seat. My line was trolling slowly behind the boat as it drifted in the breeze.

Suddenly the sound of a motor boat coming nearer intruded upon me. Noticing it was the game warden's boat, I scrambled up on the seat and started rowing rapidly toward shore. My fishing license was back in the cabin. I heard a teasing laugh and looked over my shoulder. I realized my passage was blocked by the, now quiet, motor boat with a familiar felt hat visible in the stern.

"You are Miss Welker, aren't you?" Bill asked.

"Yes, I am."

"I am the new deputy game warden. May I see your fishing license?"

"It's . . . t's up in the cabin."

"A fine alibi. Don't you know you're suppose to carry it with you always?"

"With no pockets in my shorts?"

We laughed. And then because it seemed so good to be laughing together, we laughed again. Suddenly he pretended serious.

"I'm afraid I shall have to arrest you unless you can produce your license."

"Couldn't it wait until this evening? I am having such good luck fishing now."

He considered this and finally agreed. "I'll make a special trip over tonight, but only this once. I really should take you in with me. In the future please wear shorts with pockets."

He was gone. I lay back in the boat and stared at the sky softened with clouds; little lambs with fat tails, roaming lions whose upper jaws drifted away, kangaroos with triplets in their pouches and one solitary white mountain of cotton, ponderous and round. Debussy's *clouds* over Lake Gilmore − and soon it would be moonlight . . .

The night was calm and cool and we decided to take a moonlight paddle. Our canoe had the silent, dream-like motion of a sailboat in a gentle breeze.

I thought, I will always remember the unreality of this night. It was as though I were looking through the wrong end of a telescope. This strange young man and I were small figures floating in an enormous black sea.

As I looked into the lake's dark surface, thousands of reflected stars stared back at me. Then, as I turned my face to the sky, there they were . . . crowding each other to see us. There was no border line between water and horizon, just star studded blackness and a canoe. Suddenly I was frightened.

"Bill," I asked, "What is this?"

"I don't know," he said.

I lay back against the cushions and looked at his silhouette against the stars; his hair, with ringlets each standing stubbornly distinct, his slightly prominent ears and wide strong shoulders. It was hard to be objective in such a setting.

"Are you always so serious?" he asked.

I considered this question for a moment. "Father says I have no sense of humor and perhaps he is right. Few things that amuse other people seem funny to me. But I have good times, too."

"Is this one of them?"

"Yes," I answered, almost in a whisper.

"Well, let's not work too hard at having a good time." I knew he was grinning, "Let's have fun as long as we may!"

The last phrase hit my heart like the four knocks of fate in Beethoven's Fifth. The overpowering minor melody engulfed me.

"Oh Bill, I'm afraid."

"Of what?'

"I don't know. I've never felt like this. I suppose it's because everything is strange in this half light. We are floating in the sky with the stars all around us!"

He said, "I've never met anyone like you. You say things I've always thought of but didn't know how to put into words. Other people up here never seem to feel these things, but you can."

I held out my hands to him. He took them and, coming a little closer, slowly kissed each fingertip, tenderly reassuring as though he felt my sudden panic and understood.

We beached the canoe and walked silently up the stairs. I felt sad and perplexed. We said goodnight and he was gone.

I ran upstairs to my room without speaking to my family. I threw myself upon the bed and lay there quivering. I could not understand the apprehension which overwhelmed me. Why, in something so charming, should this premonition of tragedy creep in at the very start? What did I fear? Fate seemed to be sounding drums of doom in the background of a fragile motif on the strings.

The days disappeared one after another like bright leaves falling off the trees and bringing the end of summer ever nearer. Bill and I spent our time together fishing, hiking and checking the fire lanes. We traveled through the back country's ugly burned over areas with its second growth of low scraggly scrub oaks and scrawny jackpines. This was the part of the northwoods that I could tolerate only by trying to consider its picturesque contrast to the other beauties.

Bill showed me lovely places, shyly, as though he were an artist exhibiting a new canvas to a close friend.

One of these shrines was a row of tall white birches bordering a small lake. The sun had just set and the reflection of the afterglow was gold and rose among the water reeds. We walked down to the water's edge. As always, when he showed me a new favorite spot, he searched my face for the reflection of the beauty thus revealed. My eyes were wide with delight and my lips tremulous. He quietly took me in his arms and kissed me. For ever after, that particular type of sunset evoked memories of Bill's first kiss and our silent exchange of vows.

Just before I left for Oak Park, Bill took me to the place he had reserved for last – an isolated strip of virgin forest. We had been joking as we climbed over the fence, as I had a habit of getting caught on fences. As soon as we entered the deep stillness of the woods, a sense of awe descended upon us. We walked through the tree lanes hand in hand like children. We were dwarfed by the enormous stand of white pines. The sun slanting through the dense foliage in thin shafts of golden light fell on our upturned faces.

The sound of a brook broke the silence. We searched along the deep carpet of pine needles and finally found it under an edging of tall fern. Delighted, we followed it around rocks, over logs and between miniature cliffs until it opened into a beaver pond filled with broken logs and edged irregularly with white water lilies. Now and then a large circle showed where a trout had risen for a fly. A grass covered hill led down to the dam. On it were the burned remains of a settler's cabin and a sturdy fireplace. There we ate our lunch.

Sadly, though, the beauty was marred by discord between Bill and me. The day was spent in futile arguments, always ending with the same conclusion – we could not marry. He could not ask me to live on the meager salary of a forest ranger and I could not give up my career as a doctor and disappoint my parents. The rumbling of doom reached a crescendo.

But we loved, our hearts cried, we loved! Why couldn't this summer last forever? How could we go on without each other? With the very thought of this, we held each other tight, as though nothing could ever separate us.

The shadows grew longer behind the trees. A sand piper with its strange teetering gait ran along the shore line. Soft breezes blew its footsteps away, as though it had never really been there at all. Only Bill and I were witnesses.

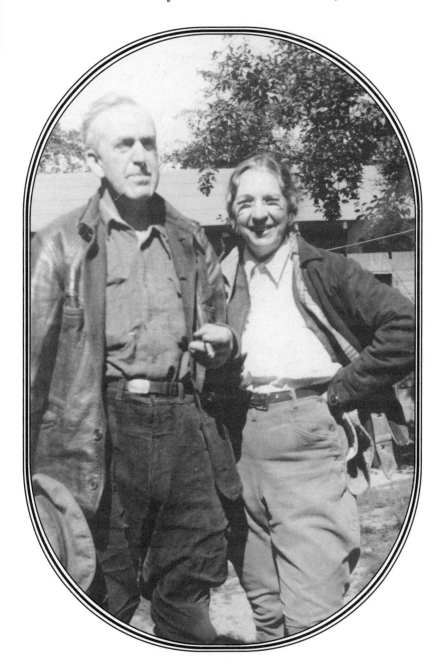

Mother and Father at Lone Larch

NEVER SAY NEVER

My nine months at home and the idyllic three months in the Northwoods were over. I would soon be returning to Cook County to finish my internship. I awaited the day a much more mature and saddened person.

Bill and I had corresponded after my return to Oak Park with letters growing more and more despairing at each exchange.

Finally one day, the last note from him arrived.

"The Bill you knew is dead," he wrote. "He walked away in the snow last night and did not come back. You must forget him."

I could not believe that perfect dream was over. I went up to my room and stayed there for several days – hardly wanting to come downstairs for meals.

Mother cooked all my favorite dishes and begged me to eat. "You will lose all the hard earned pounds you put on during this year if you don't try. How about some of these timbales? You always loved them with chicken and mushrooms."

I looked at her dear, troubled face and hated myself for hurting her. Of all the people in the world, next to Bill, I loved her the most and knew it was reciprocated. I had gone from eighty-five to one hundred and ten pounds in a year of mother's kind care and was not about to give it up now.

I made a little joke of the situation, "Boy, when I'm back eating the hospital food, I'll think of these timbales and want to run home!"

Mother laughed, "I'll have to bring you care packages from time to time, she said. And she did.

My internship resumed with Pathology under Dr. Jaffé, a pleasant, rotund Viennese with a delightful accent. He welcomed me with a warmth that helped lift my sagging ego.

"How nize to haff you with us!" he said upon my appearance in his office. "I haff great respect for your father and I'm sure you will follow in his footsteps."

I suppressed an incipient giggle at his broken English. I knew from his previous lectures that he was one of the most intellectual men I had ever met. He could take a dead patient and trace the course of his illness from the beginning to the end with logic and clarity. Most pathologists were content with making a final diagnosis by examining the affected tissue, but not Dr. Jaffé. He delved into the causes, cultured the bacteria and studied slide after slide of all the organs.

He really was a genius the way he solved these medical mysteries and I considered it a great honor to be allowed to work with him. This was not part of the regular intern program but Dr. Meyer, the Medical Administrator, had been most cordial about allowing me to make up for lost time spent in recuperating.

"You may pick any service you prefer and, since you became ill working so hard for us, we will give you six months extra credit."

I was amazed at his change of attitude for I remembered vividly how angry he had been with me over the knife-in-the-brain episode. Maybe he felt a little embarrassed about the whole thing. Anyhow, I was delighted when Dr. Meyer allowed me to spend six months with Dr. Jaffé because this was a cherished residency program and he was telling me to take it as an intern. And best of all, I would not have any night calls.

The first autopsy was traumatic. The patient was a

twenty-seven year old girl with long brown hair and a marble statue-like body. I was assigned to assist Dr. Jaffé's resident, which meant acting like a surgical nurse in an operating room. Handing instruments as needed, mopping up blood and other body fluids.

According to the patient's history she had succumbed to a particularly virulent cancer which killed her so rapidly that it hadn't distorted her appearance in any way. She hadn't even lost much weight.

I stood looking at this lovely person who was about the same age as myself and felt a great sadness for this wasted life.

I shuddered at the first long incision through the delicate white skin. Didn't the young resident mind mutilating the apparently perfect body in this way?

I asked Dr. Rosenbaum whether or not they had many such patients.

"I have never seen such a perfect specimen," he said. "What a shame she had to die, but at least she did not suffer long."

Well, I thought, here is a pathologist with compassion. So many of them, by their constant association with death and the history of long painful illnesses, become hardened to suffering. I decided I'd like to get to know him better.

The autopsy proceeded routinely with every organ riddled with the spider like growth of metastatic melanosarcome, a malignancy which had spread like a wild fire. I learned that the younger a patient, the more dangerous was the condition. I felt this internship was going to be a great learning experience.

I went back to Dr. Jaffé's office and discussed the case with him. Busy as he was, he took time to talk about this unfortunate young woman. I was very grateful.

After a month of assisting the four residents with their autopsies, I was called into Dr. Jaffé's office.

"How would you like to do all the stillborns and prematures?" he asked. "I heard that you are considering being a pediatrician, so I thought maybe this experience would be helpful."

I was thrilled and honored. I couldn't believe my fortune. "I'd like to examine these little ones. Maybe I could find out how to prevent future early deaths!"

"Splendid! That is vat Pathology is all about!" Dr. Jaffé nodded vigorously, "Otter wize, this would be a terribly sad specialty."

I did many examinations of these tiny, unfortunate creatures born before their time and was amazed at how many of them died from hemorrhages in the brain. The blood vessels were so fragile that the least pressure on their friable heads would often tear the venous channels which ran through the brain.

This was before the discovery that Vitamin K given to the mother before delivery and to the baby after delivery, could prevent many of these hemorrhages.

Occasionally, a full term newborn, either stillborn or passed away shortly after delivery, would be assigned to me — Oh, how I *wish* I could have saved these pretty little babies from their early death.

As I continued with my internship my desire to become a pediatrician became more resolute. After all, to save an octogenarian's life meant giving the person a few more years of life, but saving a baby or a child was an entirely different matter. Besides, Pediatrics was such a happy specialty, with few discouraging chronic illnesses and fewer deaths. I really was satisfied with my decision and decided to apply for a Pediatric residency. I immediately met with a rebuff from Dr. Meyer.

"My dear," he said kindly — an emotion he rarely portrayed, "I would be glad to assign you to a Pediatric residency if Dr. Blatt would approve. He is Chairman of the Pediatric Department and prides himself on never having had a woman resident." The gauntlet was thrown down.

"Well, something has to be done about that!" I said indignantly. "I know there has never been a woman surgical resident either, but I suppose it's because no one has ever fought for it and I'm going to fight for this!"

Dr. Meyer smiled, "Well, I wish you luck. Why don't you tackle the old man?"

"Will you O.K. my appointment if he agrees?"

Dr. Meyer, realizing he had painted himself into a corner, had to say, "yes."

I made an appointment via Dr. Blatt's secretary for the next day. I did not want to waste more than one sleepless night over it.

Dr. Blatt was a sixtyish, small, lean man with a stiff neck and back. He had been a career military physician and had been injured in World War I, so he had to turn halfway around to see anyone who was not immediately in front of him. He was sitting behind a huge desk and turned around part way to look at me approaching him from the side. He frowned.

"What can I do for you?" He spoke with military precision; clipped and rapid.

"I'm applying for a residency in Pediatrics starting next July First."

Dr. Blatt grunted, "Sorry, but I believe all the spaces are filled for then."

"If an opening should occur, would I be acceptable?" I asked innocently.

Dr. Blatt gave me one of those hawk-like glances that was supposed to intimidate his opponent. I had dealt with formidable males before and refused to quail.

"What you don't seem to understand is that there never has been a woman Pediatric Resident in the past and probably never will be."

"But why not? I feel that Pediatrics is a perfect specialty for a woman. Most women are fond of children and handle them beautifully."

"Then they should stay home and raise their own."

I almost laughed aloud. I'd heard that cliché so many times that it was getting to be funny. "I have spent almost nine years studying to be a doctor and I refuse to stop now because of some outworn concept that a woman's place is in the home!"

Dr. Blatt grinned ruefully.

"Touche! You have me there. I know your father well and I see he has hatched a fighting eagle."

I thanked God once more for my father.

"Dr. Meyer will approve my residency in Pediatrics if you do."

"Now, now young lady. Not so fast. I am sure my department will vote against it."

"Well, if your department agrees to it, will you accept me?"

He cleared his throat, looked at the floor, looked at the ceiling, straightened some papers on his desk and then, thinking he was safe, grudgingly said, "Yes."

I smiled triumphantly at the receptionist who had been trying to hear the rather loud conversation in the next room. I had a plan and was not going to waste any time carrying it out.

I asked for the day off from Dr. Jaffé, explaining what I wanted it for. He was most encouraging and had given me a list of the attending men on the pediatric staff. I went back to my room and grouped them according to the location of their offices.

There were ten of them scattered about the city. Three of them were on the West Side near the hospital, so that was easy. Each of them was very willing to have me as a resident, especially Dr. Henry Irish, a tall stately man with deep blue eyes and a star sapphire ring to match. He welcomed me gladly and said, "We have needed a feminine presence on the resident staff for some time."

"Three down and seven to go," I thought when I went to bed that night.

It was a little more difficult to reach the other members of the staff, since they were scattered quite widely, but I managed by the use of a borrowed car and one taxi ride.

All but one were pleasant and cooperative. The remaining doctor had been a general practitioner and, before a formal residency was required, had declared himself a Pediatrician. Whether it was because of his inadequate training or because of his upbringing in a traditional *old county* atmosphere, he was loath to accept the idea of a woman resident.

I tried all my arguments and wiles on this stubborn man without success. Suddenly I had this thought. "If all the other members of the staff voted for me, would you stand in my way?"

"No. . ." he said considering the idea and then to my surprise finished with, "If they all wanted you, I would make it unanimous." He probably thought there was no possibility that *all* of the others would vote for me and, so, felt safe in his promise.

I almost hugged him, but stopped just in time. He might think I was too forward and reverse his decision. So instead I thanked him profusely while shaking his hand over and over.

The staff meeting was the following week. Dr. Blatt called, "Order," and, after several reports, asked the residents to leave.

I was told about what happened by Dr. Irish: "Blatt said he had an embarrassing interview the previous week with an applicant for the next year's residency. He said it was a female. No one seemed surprised. He looked around and said; 'It's always been the policy of the department never to have a woman resident. We feel it might be too distracting for the male residents and also we are not too sure of the work quality. So let's have a show of hands. How many are opposed to having Dorothy Welker as a pediatric resident?'"

Irish chuckled. "You should have seen Dr. Blatt's face when not a single hand went up."

"How many were in favor?"

"All hands but one went up and when this man saw all the rest in favor his hand went up also! 'Passed unanimously!' Blatt was disgusted. Then, he said, 'Send Dr. Welker in.'"

When I returned to the staff room, Dr. Blatt growled, "Well, you asked for it! If there's trouble it's your responsibility."

I was delighted and rushed to tell Dr. Jaffé the good news.

He tilted back his chair, folded his chubby hands over his prominent abdomen and smiled. "See, I knew you could do it! In years to come there will be more and more women in professions and therefore less and less prejudice. You mark my words."

I did hug him — decorum be hanged.

The group of pathology residents I worked with the next five months, completing my internship in that department, were a close knit group who enjoyed each others' company and I was readily accepted by all. The fun and comradeship we had was a welcome relief from the handling of death everyday.

We lived in a suite of small rooms on the third floor of the old building which housed the labs. We also had one large room that housed a king-sized bed and a Steinway grand piano. Since one of the residents played, the group used to lounge around on the comfortable bed and listen quietly. After a few weeks, Dr. Rosenbaum invited me to join them. It made working with them more enjoyable because of this common bond of love for classical music.

One night after they had all retired for the evening, with Dr. Rosenbaum on that majestic bed, the other three residents were awakened by a commotion in the *music room*, as they called it.

They rushed in to find Dr. Rosenbaum grappling with a huge, black man.

"What the hell is going on here." said Dr. Hirschbaum, a young resident.

"I found this son-of-a-bitch sleeping in bed with me!," Dr. Rosenbaum, said wrathfully pointing at the now thoroughly subdued man.

"What made you come in here?" Dr. Rosenbaum asked him?

"Well, I saw the door open in the hall and this bed looked so comfortable I just had to crawl in and sleep in it. My hospital bed ain't all that soft."

"Didn't you see someone was in it?" asked Dr. Neuman, another member of the group.

"No sir, I sure didn't. It was kind of dark in here so I just crept in."

We all started to laugh except for the poor, confused man who was hustled back to his ward. Dr. Rosenbaum never lived down his reputation for being a gracious bed-mate to a wandering patient.

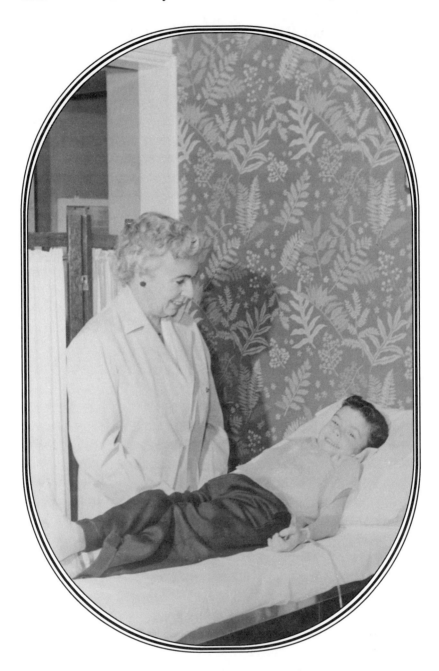

At Grant Hospital with hemophiliac patient

AN EMBARRASSING LESSON

July First came much too fast for me, for I had enjoyed the learning experience in Pathology and wished I could have stayed longer.

Dr. Jaffé offered me a complete residency of three full years because, he said, "It would take a person at least three years to scratch the surface of all there is to know about the abnormalities of the human body."

I turned it down, regretfully, because I had fought so hard to get the Pediatric Residency that I would not give it up! Knowing Dr. Blatt, I was sure he would never give me another chance.

So I kissed all my good friends and bid my teachers good-bye and went on to my next challenge.

The first obstacle I ran into was getting permission to have a room in the Children's Hospital. Again, I had to go to Dr. Blatt. He was very stuffy about it.

"You'll have to stay in the main building. I can't have you bunking with all the male residents."

I felt the color rising in my cheeks; "I wouldn't be 'bunking' as you call it with any male residents! I would merely have a room on the top floor of Children's Hospital!"

"How convenient, with seven attractive boy friends all in a row!"

"How can I travel all the way from the Seventh Floor of the old building a block away from Children's? What about the nights I'm on call?"

"A little exercise won't hurt you."

"Have you ever come across that courtyard at two in the morning? It's cold and frightening."

"What shall I tell your father if you get pregnant?" He leered at me.

"Oh, Dr. Blatt. What kind of a person do you think I am? I don't have to sit here and be insulted!" I started for the door.

Dr. Blatt looked embarrassed. "Don't get on your high horse! Come back here and sit down. I was only kidding."

That was the usual excuse for sexual harassment when the man realized he'd gone too far.

"Well, I'll make a deal with you. If you can get another woman resident to share your room, I'll consider the possibility of letting you move into *residents row*."

I agreed gladly, although I wondered whom in the world I could get.

The next day, in the large dining room for interns and residents, I saw a new woman resident. I went over and introduced myself. The woman was heavyset and muscular with a pleasant, determined expression.

"I'm the new OB and Gyne resident. I had my internship at Wesley. My name is Augusta Webster," she said.

I liked Augusta's direct manner. I felt that here was a woman I could trust; no shilly-shallying and pussy-footing around! So I came directly to the point.

"I'm in a predicament. I really want to live in Children's because all my cases are there, but the Administrator won't hear of it unless I have a woman room-mate. How would you like to join me?"

Augusta laughed, "That's the best proposition I've had today. I am crowded in with three other girls in a tiny room. Shall we go look at your space?"

So after dinner, we went over to the top floor of Children's. The room was bright and airy with twin beds and plenty of distance between two huge closets and a large bathroom with tub and shower. The windows made it quite attractive. "I feel a little guilty asking you to travel across the courtyard the nights you are on call."

"Oh, that's easy," said Augusta in an efficient manner. "I'll sleep in the nurses' dressing room if I have patients about to deliver and if I want to come back here, I'll just go through the tunnel."

I shuddered as I remembered the long winding tunnel which connected all the buildings in that square block. Not only was it very dark and lonely, but it was inhabited by a particularly nasty tribe of cats who lived on the water pipes in the ceiling and ate the rats and large water beetles which overran the place. Sometimes the mating and/or quarreling of the cats resounded throughout the long passages. Sometimes one met an intern pushing a gurney with a corpse on it for the patient's last journey to the morgue.

I looked at Augusta with great respect. What a brave woman! I felt ashamed of my own timidity, but there it was. I suppose it was due to my sheltered upbringing. Excuses? I guessed so!

Nevertheless, I was most grateful to Augusta for helping me out. She had a marvelous sense of humor. She laughed a lot and swore for emphasis. It was the start of a great friendship between two people with entirely different make ups and backgrounds.

After living a month in the bare room with curtain-less windows and white hospital spreads, I could not stand it anymore. Not knowing how Augusta would take it, I said to her one day, "How would you like it if Id dressed the room up a bit? It seems so cold and stark."

"I don't see anything wrong with it," Augusta said in a very decided manner.

"Oh, I hate it this way. If I made some nice chintz drapes with bedspreads to match, would you pay half of the cost of the material?"

Augusta shrugged, "I suppose so.   But you are so God-damned domestic!"

This statement struck me as funny and soon we were howling with laughter at the difference between us.

So the curtains were sewn, mostly through my mother's aid, and when they were hung and the bedspreads in place, Augusta had to admit they looked "OK."

I liked the place much better that way. It was more like home and if that made me seem domestic, then I guessed I was. But what was so wrong with that?

Whether it was because the room seemed cozy or whether the other residents liked Augusta and my jolly company, Room 707 became a hangout for most of the other residents when they were off duty.

I especially liked the head resident, an older, married man, Dr. O'Brien, who had been in general practice for twenty years before he decided to become a Pediatrician. He was kind and understanding, a pleasant contrast to Dr. Blatt's authoritative stance. He also knew many practical diagnostic points about infants' and children's illnesses which he shared with me and the other residents.

Some of these younger men were scornful of his *old fashioned methods*. All they wanted to do was a complete laboratory work up before they bothered to do a physical examination, an opinion which bothered me. I had been indoctrinated by Dr. Chauvet, Father's friend. He had taught me that, next to a thorough history, a complete physical examination was of the greatest importance in diagnosing a case.

Unfortunately, the lesson was learned at the expense of my dignity − an embarrassing incident in Dr. Chauvet's physical diagnosis class. The students were learning how to examine each other. The four girls were in one examining room and the rest of the Section in the other examining rooms.

The girls pulled straws for being the patient and I was *it*. I had to strip to the waist but forgot to remove my bead choker. The girls were listening to my heart and lungs with their new stethoscopes when in walked Dr. Chauvet followed by his intern. I nearly fell off the table when I recognized Jim Scully, a boy with whom I had several dates. What made it worse was he was blushing more than I was. He looked everywhere except at *the patient.*

Dr. Chauvet, completely oblivious to what was going on, demonstrated the art of percussion on my bare back. Jim looked out the window.

"Now a hollow sound," said Dr. Chauvet, "means there is air in the lung. And a dull sound means there is consolidation there, such as pneumonia or fluid. It is very important to differentiate the kinds of pitch." He knocked on a table to demonstrate a solid structure sound.

I prayed he would leave shortly, which he did, followed closely on his heels by Jim.

The girls who had hardly been able to contain their giggles burst into loud laughter as soon as the door was closed. I grabbed my brassiere and blouse and hurriedly put them on.

"You beasts!" I said, "You can practice on yourselves! I'm leaving."

A week later, I met Jim in the hall on the way to another class. He apologized, "I'm so sorry about what happened last week with Dr. Chauvet. I had no idea he was going into the girls' examining room. I guess he never gave it a thought."

"Well, maybe he didn't, but I certainly did," I said. "I was horrified when I saw you."

It was very gentlemanly of Jim to apologize instead of letting that embarrassment hang between us. I accepted his apology and liked him all the better for it.

As awful as the whole incident was, I completely agreed with Dr. Chauvet on the importance of a thorough examination.

I decided the propensity for relying on lab work was sheer laziness on the part of some of the residents. It was so much easier to write an order for a chest X-ray than to painstakingly go over a chest inch by inch with observation, palpation, percussion and auscultation. True, X-ray was a valuable tool, but only as an adjunct, I thought. The whole process might take longer but it was much more accurate.

Dr. O'Brien approved of my conscientiousness and, during rounds, demonstrated to the other residents how often this system paid off in correct diagnosis.

The tragic part of it was that it did not help much in treatment. In the 1930's, very few antibiotics were available. I hated to come down to the infant pneumonia ward in the mornings because so many of the children had died during the night.

Years later, as an attending physician I made rounds in this same ward and thanked God for penicillin which cut down the mortality rate from pneumonia in infants under one year from 20% to 2%.

DR. BLATT'S SIDE SHOWS

Dr. Blatt's rounds were spoken of with trepidation throughout the whole Cook County Hospital. They were known as "Blatt's Side Shows," the point of them being to show up the unfortunate intern or resident whose case it was.

He appeared at seven o'clock on Mondays and Thursdays and heaven help any member of the house staff who was not in the doctors' room to meet him! He'd look around with his hawk-like grim glance and say, "Where's Ferguson? – Or Riley – Or Sharp?" as the case might be. "Suffering from a hangover? Oh, there you are . . . I thought you had died."

There were always small, subdued chuckles from this audience who knew he liked to have his humor appreciated.

I never laughed at his cruel remarks and, in punishment, he always gave me his doctor's bag to carry.

"Here you are, Doctor," he'd say handing it to me, "make yourself useful."

I would have loved to give him a snippy reply, but I did not quite dare to do it. Besides, I thought it would have afforded him too much pleasure to know he could get a rise out of me. He tried his best to make life so miserable for me that I would have to quit, then he could carry out his boast of never having had a woman complete her Pediatric Residency.

He was particularly malicious in his rounds on my cases, so I prepared them meticulously, anticipating any questions he might ask.

A typical case presentation would go as follows: Dr. Blatt and his huge entourage of white uniformed followers, interns, residents, an occasional attending man, plus a nurse or two, would come swooping into a particular ward. They would approach a bedside and he would ask, "Whose case is this?"

The resident involved would step forward and hand him the chart. Then the inquisition would begin.

"What kind of hand writing is this?" he'd demand. "I can't read a word of it! Tell me about this case."

The resident would start in a soft voice.

"Speak up, man. I can't hear you when you mumble."

And so it went, with everyone becoming more and more uncomfortable, especially the unfortunate resident. This was Colonel Blatt's army training showing through and nobody liked it, least of all, me, still, impatiently, carrying his Doctor's bag.

I was always glad when none of my cases were on the agenda and particularly happy when I could discuss Dr. Blatt's antics with Dr. O'Brien.

"Why does he have to be so mean?" I asked Dr. O'Brien in private.

"Because he's a homely, little man and has to make up for his physical inferiority by pushing his subordinates around," Dr. O'Brien speculated. "In fact, he's turned out to be a 100% bastard. Don't pay any attention to him."

"That's pretty hard to do, especially when I'm toting his bag for him."

"You are a bit down, aren't you?" asked Dr. O'Brien sympathetically.

"Not just a bit," I answered. "What can I do about it?"

"Well, I have just the prescription for that! Golf."

"I've never played it in my life!"

"All the better. So you'll learn and it surely will take your mind off of Dr. Blatt and his dastardly deeds. Get yourself an inexpensive set of five clubs and a cloth golf bag and meet me at the back parking lot tomorrow at five a.m."

I spent my lunch hour shopping for golf equipment and was all ready to go the next morning.

There was Dr. O'Brien with two other favorite residents of Dr. O'Brien's and a car borrowed from the only resident who owned one. Everyone was on a tight budget, since no one received a salary in those days.

We drove out to Northwestern Golf Course, an interesting, forest-lined, municipal golf course with mostly par three and par four holes – a great place for beginners.

Dr. O'Brien taught me how to approach the ball on the tee. "Head down, left elbow straight, an overlapping grip and a smooth follow through." I had a terrible habit of lifting my head to see where the ball was going to go.

"Don't lift your head up!" Dr. O'Brien bellowed. "Why can't you remember that? You'll hook or slice into the rough every time or even top the ball, which is worse because it won't go anywhere if you do that!"

"I do think I could throw the ball farther than I can hit it with a driver," I complained.

"Now, don't get discouraged," said Dr. Perry Sharp, a former football player. "I had the same trouble when I was starting out." And then he hit a beautiful straight drive two hundred yards down the fairway.

"Oh, do you think I'll ever be able to do that?" I asked Dr. O'Brien.

He laughed, his Irish eyes full of mischief.

"Oh, maybe by the time you're a hundred."

I trudged on to where my ball was hidden in the rough.

"Throw it out. You'll never be able to get it out of there." said Perry. "We won't watch you."

"Is it against the rules?" I asked innocently.

"Oh, no." the other three answered tongue in cheek. So I threw it out. Years later, I would be penalized for doing that because I honestly believed it was allowed.

I liked to make short chip shots onto the green. They were so easy and did not require any strength. Putting too, was fun. I became quite adept at a one putt score, if the ball was not more than twenty feet away from the hole.

The two residents and Dr. O'Brien took great pride in my low scores, made that way mostly because of my accurate putting and approach shots. But they moaned with mock horror at my impossible tee shots.

Nevertheless these early morning games really helped break the monotony of the hard work in the regular wards and in the Emergency Ward, where, like all the residents and interns in other services, we had to take turns for night services.

Emergency was a real contrast to the comparative quiet of the Pediatric Ward and Newborn Nursery. The Ward was in a large section on the first floor of the new building and it was constantly busy, day and night. A shooting, or any accident, was immediately brought in by the police. Many of these patients were DOA, dead on arrival. I had not had this service as an intern and was horrified at all the tragedies I was exposed to there.

Miss Burkholder, the cynical, bored, night nurse in charge, had "seen everything," as she said, and this was not an idle boast. She gave directions like a top sergeant to all the interns and residents who worked there, because she knew more about handling trauma cases than did most of them.

The one person I really respected was the Night Medical Superintendent, Roger Gilquist. His opinion was only called for when a serious condition that required surgery. The rest of the time, he sat with his feet propped on his desk reading medical journals. Woe to the intern or resident who disturbed his studies! They were treated to the third degree.

After the unfortunate bearer of bad news had shifted uneasily from one foot to the other for many minutes, the dragon raised his shaggy head.

"Yes, what is it this time?"

"We have a very serious case, sir."

"I know. They are all serious at this time of night — or they better be!"

The intern gulped, "I really think this one calls for an operation."

"Oh, you do, do you? What's the history?"

The history was given and then Doctor Gilquist asked appropriate questions, "Any rebound tenderness? Rectal exam? Temperature? White count? Differential? X-ray findings? Urine?"

If any of these were missing or equivocal, the intern was sent back for further details.

It was only after Dr. Gilquist was completely satisfied with the work up and intelligence of the intern that he slowly took his feet down and said, "See you in the operating room."

Once there, he examined the patient, studied the chart carefully and only then told the anesthetist to proceed. If Dr. Gilquist operated on a patient, he or she really needed the procedure. But he was quite skilled and carefully instructed the intern and resident in the technique of the surgery. It made up for the uncomfortable moments in his office.

If the patient brought into the Emergency Room merely needed first aid, Dr. Gilquist was not disturbed. The first night I was given a suturing job on Maggie, a pretty black girl of about eighteen. She had many knife slashes on her face and arms.

I was shocked at the damage and asked, "Who did this to you?"

"My boyfriend."

It was always the same answer. I wondered after this experience how the boy friend could still be the friend. He surely wouldn't be my boyfriend anymore if he assaulted me. I remembered giving back Doc's pin for just a slap. I certainly would never be battered, at least not more than once.

Miss Burkholder complimented me on my neat repair of all those cuts. She shook her head with disgust at the black girl's attitude.

"We see so many women here who have been beaten over and over again. I give some of them pep talks but it doesn't seem to do any good. They seem to enjoy having their boyfriends or husbands maul them about. I'd never put up with that kind of crap."

And I, looking at her fierce expression and strong muscles, believed her.

"Why don't you go into surgery?" asked Miss Burkholder. "You seem to have the knack of it."

"I like to do things with my hands," I said, "but I can't take worrying about the patient afterwards."

"I think that's an asset. Too many surgeons feel when they are finished closing up that it's the resident's responsibility from then on. I'd like to see a few more of them sit up all night with dangerous, post-operative cases. There are exceptions, of course," Miss Burkholder admitted grudgingly. She hated to give compliments even in her thoughts. That was why I appreciated the remarks she made about my stitching technique.

I asked my patient to return in five days so that I personally could remove the stitches and, incidentally, monitor the results. I was especially anxious to see how the subcutaneous horse hair stitches would work on the pretty girl's face.

"But," I warned her, "If you go back to that horrible creep, don't come back to me. Someone else can remove your stitches."

The girl smiled and left after getting a tetanus shot. She seemed to mind that more than any suturing, probably because of the local anesthetic I was careful to give before sewing.

Many car and motorcycle accidents came into Emergency and I was impressed by the efficient way Miss B got the Orthopedic Residents and attending men to function. Those cases received prompt and excellent care and most of them were admitted to Orthopedic Wards or, if they had head injuries, to the Neurological service. Unfortunately, many of them were so badly injured that they succumbed no matter what heroic care was given to them. I began to understand why Miss B looked so cynical and tired.

"It must be wearing to see this kind of thing night after night." I said to Miss B while we were having one of our rare coffee breaks.

Miss B sipped her hot coffee slowly, "Yes, I sometimes wonder why I do it. This is my twentieth year here and every pay-day I think I'll hand in my notice, but I never do. I'm afraid life would be pretty dull anywhere else. Besides I like to take some of the conceit out of these dumb interns. They think they know it all, but when I get through with them, they're not so sure. That's the first step toward becoming a good doctor."

I looked at Miss B and realized, perhaps, she was not so cynical after all.

Maggie, the little black girl, came back promptly five days later and, when her stitches were removed, looked almost pretty again.

"Well, what about the boy friend?" I asked with Miss B as an interested bystander.

"That black gorilla?" she answered. "I'll spit in his eye if he ever comes around again?"

We were delighted. Maybe this was one battered female we had converted.

Of all the cases I encountered in the Emergency Ward, the suicide attempts were the hardest for me to take. So many of these unfortunates were in their late teens or early twenties. They seemed so young and vulnerable, unable to take the stresses of life.

One handsome, twenty-year-old man had taken over a hundred mercuric chloride tablets, usually used as an antiseptic, which he had filched from the drug store where he worked. His kidneys shut down completely and he was in critical condition.

I worked on him all that night. He recovered by some miracle, aided by the prompt pumping out of his stomach plus an antidote intravenously and peritoneal effusion. I went to see him in Male Medicine each day during the following weeks. When he was released he came to say good-bye, but not to thank me. Instead he said, "Well Doc, I'm leaving now, but you could have saved all your time and effort, because I'm going out and do it all over again!"

It had been a long night and day on the pediatric ward and I was in no mood for such nonsense. "OK, if that's the way you want it, do as you like. But I'm telling you right now, don't come back to me when I'm on the night shift of Emergency because I won't admit you."

The young man's eyes opened up wide and his self pitying expression changed to one of amazed acceptance. He was quiet for a few minutes and then asked, "Do you have the name of a shrink that could get me out of this mess?"

I wrote a small note of introduction to Dr. Lane, one of the few sensible and compassionate psychiatrists I knew.

Dear Chuck,
Please help this man. He's worth saving.
Thanks, Dorothy.

I sealed it in an envelope and wrote Dr. Charles Lane's address and telephone number on the outside.

"Call him up now and tell his receptionist I am referring you to him. Don't let her put you off. If you have any trouble seeing him, let me know."

The defeated look in his eyes changed to a more hopeful expression and perhaps showed even a touch of gratitude.

After he left, I thought, using one of Charlie's Yiddish expressions, "Well I do believe that was my *mitzvah* for the day."

MARRIED MEN AND MORAL DILEMMAS

As the time neared to begin our next services, I asked Dr. O'Brien when he was going to announce assignments.

"Why?" he asked, "Is there anyone you would particularly prefer?"

"I'd really like the Tuberculosis Ward." This was one of the most sought after services of the Pediatric Residency because it was headed by Dr. Joseph Greengard, a serious physician, the youngest member of the attending staff.

Dr. O'Brien smiled and said, "You really know how to pick 'em. All the nurses around here are crazy about Dr. Greengard."

"It's the service I want, not the man!" After I worked with Dr. Greengard for a few weeks I was no longer so sure.

I found him reserved in a charming sort of way. I thought he looked like Ronald Coleman, only more handsome, since his nose was not as large as that of the British actor. But he had the same dignified look and the same gallant way of walking.

One day, I asked the middle-aged Charge Nurse, Miss Jenkins, whether or not he was married.

She answered swiftly, "Oh yes, didn't you know?"

I sighed, "Why was it that all the cute ones were married? In my naïveté, I believed the nurse. I didn't know at the time that Miss Jenkins had quite a crush on her attending man, so she was not about to tell me that he was single. She had even named her demonstration doll Josephine, much to the amusement of the student nurses she taught.

"Now I'll show you how to take Josephine's auxiliary temperature," she said causing many suppressed smiles from the girls. Or, "I'm going to show you the proper way to bathe *Josephine*." There was even more obvious amusement from the student nurses. To think Miss Jenkins had the temerity to name a plastic doll after the austere Dr. Greengard was just too much.

"The poor old thing," everyone whispered, "She has no one else to love."

She didn't know what a huge favor she'd done by making me think Dr. Greengard was married. I didn't know it, but he was one of the most sought after bachelors on the North Side of Chicago among the Jewish mamas. A doctor in his early thirties and handsome in addition! So he received many dinner invitations to meet the unmarried daughters, and he was uncomfortably aware that his *previous engagement* excuses were seen as obviously false.

I was respectfully polite when we made rounds on the ward and listened attentively to his diagnostic and treatment regimens. Thinking he was married, I was careful not to be overly friendly. Of course, I had no idea that he was weary of being pursued by mothers and daughters intent on marriage. My reserved manner, being the exact opposite, was piquing his interest.

So as the two month's TB service came to a close, Joseph and I were talking over cases in the doctors' lounge, when suddenly he said, "There will be an especially good program at the Chicago Symphony tonight. How would you like to go?"

"With you?" I asked, surprised.

"With me, of course. Why not?"

"I'm sorry, but I never date married men."

There was a startled moment of silence and then Dr. Greengard said, "Married, hell! I've never even been engaged!"

I could not believe it. Suddenly I saw Miss Jenkins' sad face.

"But. . . I thought . . . I was told . . . " I stammered.

"By whom?"

I did not answer. I could not give away the poor old maid's secret. "It's no matter. I'd love to attend the concert with you." And that was the truth.

He called for me at seven-thirty in front of the grayish white formal structure which had played and would continue to play an important role in our lives, the Children's Division of the Cook County Hospital.

The evening was a delight. We discovered that Bach and Mozart were our favorites and late Bartok and some Stravinsky set our teeth on edge, although early Bartok and many Stravinsky compositions sent our spirits soaring. We especially loved Debussey. During intermission, our conversation was about medicine and music.

"Well, how did it go?" asked Augusta from her bed when I returned to my room.

"Oh, it was divine! I haven't had such a satisfying evening in a long time."

"Any passes?"

"Augusta! From Dr. Greengard? Of course not. He was a perfect gentleman."

"Oh heck!" said Augusta and she turned over and went to sleep.

I did not get much rest that night. Strains of Bach and Debussey kept resounding in my thoughts. I made a resolution to be careful and not ruin my chances. I had obtained a nibble by playing it cool and was not about to let the fish get away by pulling in the line too soon.

But I wondered what he was really like under that almost British exterior. Was he cold to the core or were there fires burning as in the center of the earth? Could a hidden volcano suddenly erupt? The possibilities were exciting to contemplate – no wonder I couldn't sleep!

Had he enjoyed the evening as much as I? He seemed less

withdrawn. Would he ask me out again now that I'd be in a different ward? I really hoped so. The only chance to see him again was at the next staff meeting, about three weeks away. It seemed a long time to wait, but somehow I felt it sure it was against his customary mode of action to make an obvious move.

Sure enough, nothing happened for three weeks. For the staff meeting, I put on a brand new white uniform with starched jacket and a bright red handkerchief peeking out of the breast pocket. It was not my usual apparel but I felt happy and wanted to share my joy with the world.

"Well," said Augusta as she saw me leave, "you're really dressed up fancy! I wonder what fish that bait is supposed to catch?"

I blushed. "Oh Augusta, you're the limit! I'm just tired of the old uniforms. I thought I'd put on something fresh for a change."

"That hankie is surely *fresh* all right. I hear that bright red is one of the favorite colors for fishing lures." I closed the door on Augusta's cackling laugh.

Many of the staff were assembled in the doctors' lounge and the air was hazy with tobacco smoke. I sat in the front row because most of the other seats were taken. I was surprised at how fast my heart was beating.

Dr. Blatt rapped for order, his head tilted to the side and his back rigid as usual. I wished I could get over my intense dislike of him. The minutes of the last meeting were read and approved, a few reports were given by various residents.

Then Dr. Blatt called on me, "I'm sure Dorothy has something to say, haven't you, my dear? Women always do."

I stood up as I had always been taught to do when addressing my elders. My cheeks were as red as my handkerchief. I did have something important to discuss.

"I would like to ask a hypothetical question. If an attending man requests a resident to perform a procedure which the resident believes would jeopardize the patient's life, can the resident refuse?"

There was a disapproving silence – then several indignant voices were raised simultaneously.

"The idea!"

"No attending man would suggest such a thing."

"Just like a woman!"

I sat down amidst all the uproar. I had no idea I would stir up such a commotion.

Dr. Blatt rapped loudly for order. "One at a time, please, gentlemen. One at a time."

Dr. Steward, the one doctor beside Dr. Blatt who had been the most reluctant to accept me as a resident, uncrossed his legs and muttered through his cigar. "I don't believe there is one of us here who would suggest such a procedure. What is this all about?" He glared fiercely at me, his expression suggesting he had not wanted to approve of me a few months previously and certainly did not approve of me now. I was sure he felt vindicated in his first opinion of me.

"May I answer that?" I asked Dr. Blatt.

"If you like."

First of all, I must tell you that it is not a hypothetical situation and the attending man is not here today. This was on the Premature Service and the person requesting this research is an associate who has only recently been appointed to the staff."

"What was the purpose of the research?" Dr. Blatt asked.

"It was to determine whether the spinal fluid was similar to the cisternal fluid in a normal preemie and also in one with meningitis or one with blood in the ventricles."

"You mean you had to do both a spinal and a cisternal puncture on each premature chosen for the experiment?" asked Dr. Greengard. He seemed shocked at the idea.

I answered eagerly. "That was what bothered me. These preemies have enough trouble without adding unnecessary traumas to their existence."

"What was the purpose of this experiment?" asked Dr. O'Brien.

"To determine whether there was a blockage of fluid in ventricular hemorrhage or meningitis."

"Did you perform this procedure on any of them?" Dr. Blatt asked sternly.

"I had done a spinal on a meningitis case and I was just about to insert the cisternal needle in the base of the skull when I could not do it. I remembered Dr. Jaffé saying, 'In a two thousand gram premature there is only two millimeters distance between the covering of the cisterna magna and the medulla oblongata where the respiratory center is located. Go just a shade too far and you will have a dead premature.' So I could not do it," I explained.

"Did you inform the associate that you deliberately disobeyed his orders?" Dr. Blatt asked, revealing, as usual, his military background.

"Yes, I did."

"And what did he say?"

"He was very angry so I told him that I could not take the responsibility of possibly killing all those preemies and if he wanted to undertake the experiment, he could do the cisternal punctures himself. He then said he would report my insubordination to you, Dr. Blatt."

"Which he did, " said Dr. Blatt. "That is why I called on you. I asked him to come today and bring it up at this meeting. but I notice he is conspicuous by his absence. How about some discussion of this case? You may leave if you wish, Dorothy."

"Do I have to?" I meekly asked.

"No, if you have the desire to stay, you may. But I warn you, it might not be pleasant." I stayed and the discussion was heated. Some of the men felt that this action was setting a precedent of disobedience among the interns and residents.

Dr. Stewart led the hew and cry. It reminded me of a fox hunt with the dogs baying at the fleeing animal, but, by golly, I was not trying to escape. I would turn on the pack and stand my ground.

"Why didn't you come to me with this matter sooner?" asked Dr. Blatt, frowning.

How could I answer that? If I told the truth I would have said, "Because I knew you would have been only too happy to suspend me for insubordination without even bringing it up at a staff meeting." Instead I answered, "This only happened late yesterday and I did not want to bother you at home last night. I thought it could wait for this morning's staff meeting."

A welcome murmur of approval reached my ears. "Now we're getting somewhere," I thought.

Dr. Blatt turned his body in my direction. He looked as though he had suddenly realized that the fox was more intelligent than he had thought.

"Well, is there more discussion before we have a vote?"

Dr. Greengard stood up. He did not look in my direction, but I could feel friendliness towards me.

"I thoroughly approve of Dr. Welker's actions. I would have done the same thing if I had been ordered to do this procedure. I feel the knowledge gained is not worth the risk entailed."

The staff listened intently to his words for they valued his opinion. In the past, his recommendations had been accepted by the majority.

"Any more discussion? Well, if not, I shall ask Dr. Welker and the other residents to leave while we take the vote as to Dr. Welker's possible suspension."

I walked out of the meeting with my head held high, but once outside I didn't feel so brave. I sat on the bench outside the door, wondereding what I would do if the staff suspended me. The other residents smiled at me and went to their respective wards.

Well, I was not through fighting yet! I'd take it to the discipline committee and, if necessary, to Dr. Meyer. I thought he would back me up, since he had been so understanding about my illness. But nevertheless, I did some serious praying:

"Please God," I prayed. "Don't let them suspend me. I really did it to save those preemies lives."

The time dragged on — ten, fifteen, twenty minutes. I imagined Dr. Stewart squinting through his cigar smoke and making cynical remarks. I knew it would really come down to a battle between him and Dr. Greengard with Dr. Blatt tilting the scales against me.

The door opened and Dr. Blatt asked me to come back for the verdict. As I resumed my seat, I felt as though I were a prisoner on the dock. My cheeks were more flushed than ever.

"I am required to inform you that you may continue your residency," he said. However, because of the unique circumstances, we will transfer you to another service. That is all."

I arose and started to leave but before I reached the door I turned and said to the staff, who were watching me closely, "Thank you, so much. I really appreciate your decision."

Later, I met Dr. Greengard for lunch in the dining room. I asked, "What happened after I left the meeting?"

He smiled, "What goes on there is strictly confidential but I will tell you this, you had plenty of supporters. Personally, I think that was an unwise request on the associate's part."

"I can't thank you enough for backing me up. I really was terrified that I'd be suspended."

"I know how you must have felt. But it was such an unfair request that no one should have agreed to it."

I looked down at my plate and thought what an honorable man he was. I hoped he would ask me out again!

As though he read my mind, Dr. Greengard said, "I have two Chicago Symphony concert tickets for next Thursday. It looks like a pretty good program. Would you like to go with me?"

I laughed, "Oh, I never date married men!" I teased, remembering my boner of the first time he had invited me out.

He thought that was funny too, so he answered as he had before. "Married, hell! Why I've never even been engaged."

So the date was set and we enjoyed many pleasant evenings after that.

ROMANCE AT THE WORLD'S FAIR

The year of residency went past far too quickly with a great deal of acquired practical knowledge, thanks to several of the attending men, associates and Dr. O'Brien. I often thought about what he had said when I was playing golf. "I may not have taught you a great deal of pediatrics, but you will remember me when you have a golf club in your hand." I remembered him for both.

It was a sad day when all the residents met in Augusta's and my room for a good-bye party. We did a lot of reminiscing about the past year, remembering many interesting cases and, of course, our brilliant diagnoses and successful treatment of them.

We laughed at the memory of how the huge, hard drinking, naked buddy had romped around the sun deck. He was pounding his heavy chest and crying, "Me Tarzan! Where's Jane?" It had taken four residents to hog-tie him and lock him in his room from which they had heard the Tarzan yell far into the night.

But, the most amusing of all was finding the shyest resident holed up in a linen closet with a pretty young student nurse, locked in a passionate embrace. We told him he was not acting so shy then!

We sadly said good-bye, all leaving the next morning for far flung practices, and we promised solemnly to keep in touch. At least we knew we would see each other once a year at the American Academy of Pediatrics Annual meeting. That made me feel better.

My colleagues couldn't resist teasing me about my *boyfriend* Dr. Greengard.

"Why did you have to pick an old man? Why not one of us young whippersnappers?" They asked. "When are you getting married?"

I felt very uncomfortable at all this kidding so I answered indignantly, "First of all, he is only six and a half years older than I am. And besides, we've never even discussed marriage. He is a confirmed bachelor."

"I bet his mother would not let him marry a Gentile," said Ruby, one of the Jewish residents.

"You are cruel, all of you," I said, "and I hope you all marry hideous, rich, older women who will hen-peck you to death!"

They loved that because they realized their barbs had really hit home.

The saddest parting was with Augusta, who was continuing her OB & Gyne residency. She was a very deft surgeon with enough emotional stability to withstand the trauma of post-operative occurrences.

We packed up our possessions and I presented Augusta with the chintz curtains and spreads so her new room back in the old building would not look so stark. "Not that you'd care — you ungrateful wretch!" I taunted her for her attitude. "But I would hate to think of you living in a slum. Besides I don't know what I'd do with them in Oak Park."

"Oh," said Augusta. "Just to salve your tender sensibilities I'll take them, but you'll have to hang them up for me because I know I'll never get around to it!"

So nothing would do but that I got several of the residents to help cart the spreads and drapes over to Augusta's new room and deck it out.

"There you are." I said to her, "Think of me when you are especially un-domestic."

"Thank you very much." said she sarcastically. "I will think of you when I go to sleep among all this interior design splendor."

My greatest uncertainty was whether or not I would ever see Joseph Greengard again. We had exchanged telephone numbers and I mentioned that I was going to spend the summer working in a booth of the University College of Medicine at the World's Fair. It sounded like fun.

"I doesn't sound too appealing to me," said Joseph, "All those people milling about and asking stupid questions."

"But I like people, " I answered. It reminded me of a remark of Mother's, "If I had my 'druthers' I'd have an apartment with a big bay window at State and Lake where I could sit and watch the people go by."

I supposed Mother and I were both extroverts and most extroverts like mingling with people while introverts are all surrounded with a little shell, like a snail, and only poke their heads out to eat.

I guessed Joseph was an introvert, although he loved his patients and seemed extroverted enough with them. He had once said, "I would be very happy being a pediatrician if it weren't for the mothers!"

I had seen his tenderness with children. He was fond of all of them and they sensed it. So he had no trouble gaining their confidence. He could do anything with them and they'd just look up and smile. I learned the technique of handling my patients from him. The main component of a painless examination was love. Also, he was perfectly honest with them.

If they asked him "Will it hurt?" he would say, "Just a little bit." Or if it would be very painful he's say, "It will hurt quite a lot but just for a minute!" He earned their trust in that way and Dr. Greengard's little patients always believed him.

Yes, I wondered If I'd ever see this admirable man again. I

didn't know the surprise in store for me while I worked at the exciting Chicago World's Fair.

I was in charge of handing out health pamphlets explaining the services of the outpatient clinics of the College of Medicine. I liked to see the pleased expressions on many of the faces of the poor when they realized there was someplace for them to go.

I demonstrated, over the loud speakers, the effect of holding one's breath on the heart rate. It was called *Sinus Arrhythmia*, and was usually restricted to children. If they breathed fast, their hearts went faster and if they held their breath, their hearts slowed down.

I positioned a stethoscope connected to a microphone over my left chest and held my breath. The steady klop-klop of my heart beat became less frequent and when I breathed rapidly it speeded up. I always had an interested little group of people gathered around me for each showing. They were amazed.

After each demonstration I always asked whether there were any questions.

I was embarrassed when a voice I recognized said, very professionally, "Doctor, how do you account for the fact that you have sinus arrhythmia when it usually occurs only in children and adolescents?"

I looked around and saw him, handsome and impeccably dressed as usual, standing way back at the edge of the crowd. I stuttered, "I really cannot explain it, Doctor. I've always had it."

"Could it be that you are an arrested adolescent?"

The audience laughed, but I did not. However, my pique rapidly disappeared at my pleasure of seeing Joseph again.

"Well, I had a time finding this booth," he said. "This is some spread."

"I know, I was late for the first performance because I couldn't find the booth either, even with a map. Of course I've never had any sense of direction. Father always said, 'If Dorothy wants to go right when she is driving and comes to a crossroads, she should turn left and she will be going correctly.'"

Joseph smiled, his hazel eyes glanced at me in a way I had only seen him look at children.   Maybe there was some advantage in being an arrested adolescent.   He had always teased me about my childlike penmanship and I had always countered, "You are just envious because no one can decipher anything you write."

So now that he had found me, we spent all his Wednesday afternoons off and two or three evenings a week enjoying the fair.

There were a dozen ethnic restaurants, many of which had pleasant appropriate dance music.   I found to my disappointment that Joseph was not a good dancer.   He tried but just did not have the knack.   He said, "A good dancer is a sign of a misspent youth!"   That was blasphemy to me, having taught ballroom dancing in college.

But this fit in with his studious personality.   Medicine had been his goal ever since high school and he had not seen the necessity of wasting time on girls and such trivialities as dating and dancing.   So we sat and talked through many interesting dinners, and all the while, under the table, my rebellious feet kept time to the music.

The Shakespeare plays were our greatest delight.   An entire company of actors from the Globe Theatre in London had been imported for the World's Fair and they performed a different play every night.   Joseph, who was quite a Shakespearean buff, would explain the plot of the evening's performance during dinner.   The actors were experts and it was a pleasure to listen to their British diction.   I enjoyed myself immensely.

Soon, instead of two or three evenings a week Joseph came out almost every night.   I wondered what was happening to his practice.   He must have found obliging friends to fill in for him.

It was a long way on the "L" from the South Side by the lake to the western suburb of Oak Park.   It was convenient for me to have Joseph drive me home every night.   During those night drives, we began to explore each other's beliefs, points of view, backgrounds and family ties.

I told him I was the only child of an only child – well practically because my mother's older sister had died before she was born. I told him about my mother's mother, who was a very strong-minded woman. She also had a peculiarly insensitive streak in her nature.

My mother, Evie, was a lovely soft spoken child. When Mother would walk with Grandmother down the main street, many people would stop and admire her for her large brown eyes and long dark hair. They would say, "What a beautiful child!" and Mrs. Hutchinson would say, "Do you think she's pretty? You should have seen her sister!" I told Joseph that I cringed whenever I thought of that remark.

Many other intimacies were exchanged. Joseph told me that he was the middle child of five in an orthodox Jewish family. His older brother had died of encephalitis, contracted while he had attended the University of Illinois, Urbana-Champaign. Therefore, his father refused to send Joseph to college, thinking that his beloved eldest son would still have been alive if he had not gone there.

Joseph, who had always wanted to be a doctor, had to work his way through college and medical school taking a year off in the process. He said, "It was grim. I was a delivery boy, a cigar factory worker, a librarian's assistant and a taxi driver among other things. I wouldn't have minded so much if my father didn't couldn't afford it."

"A taxi-driver! Now I know why you drive the way you do."

He looked at me sideways out of his almond shaped eyes.

"Is that supposed to be a joke?"

"No, not at all. I have to close my eyes sometimes when you duck between cars on the outer drive."

"I'm sorry if I scare you, but you don't have to worry. I've never had an accident."

I wanted to say, "But there's always a first time." But I did not, because I was still a little in awe of this learned man whom I had heard give such brilliant lectures.

Inevitably, we came to discussions of each other's religious beliefs.

My family was originally Pennsylvania Dutch Reformed but there were no Dutch Reformed churches in Oak Park or Chicago, except for one on the South Side. We attended the First Presbyterian Church of Oak Park, but never joined it. I had always felt that both Mother and Father were truly religious in belief, even though they did not go to church regularly. Moreover, they accepted all other beliefs with great tolerance.

Joseph, however, had trouble with his family's religion. He had been forced to attend Hebrew school every weekday afternoon following grammar school much to his disgust. The Greengards lived in an old-fashioned house on the outskirts of Chicago. This was located in an Irish Catholic neighborhood and Joseph had many friends there.

He was an excellent athlete and enjoyed playing baseball and football with the boys in the corner lot. So he resented not being able to play with them as much as he wanted because his parents required him to go to Hebrew school. He was teased unmercifully by his peers, in fact he became so bitter about it that, once he was on his own, he never attended synagogue services again.

The old adage, *You can lead a horse to water, but you can't make him drink,* really was appropriate in his case. I was sorry for him because he seemed to be without a religion.

He denied this, "I believe there is a Divine Power but not a personal God who answers one's prayers. I think God is purpose and order to the universe. What physician would deny that, knowing the marvelous complexities of the body's physiology?"

So I had to be satisfied with that. In a way, it was better if Joseph did not have a firm connection with an organized religion and also that my parents were not pillars of the Presbyterian church. What a conflict that would have been!

I was happier than I had been for a long time; ever since my idyllic episode with Bill. However, this was different, more stable with so many interests in common. It was reality, fastened to the ground, as opposed to fantasy floating in the clouds.

Joseph and I were growing closer. I invited him to Sunday dinner in Oak Park after the Fair had closed. He accepted reluctantly. He had been bored by too many family dinners.

But he did not appear to be bored at this one, probably because my father was unusually cordial. He remembered Joseph as having been one of his most brilliant students, which made him tops as far as Father was concerned.

Mother was quiet as usual. Nanny, my Grandmother Hutchinson, was interested in all Joseph's remarks and Aunt Alice, father's older sister kept looking down shyly most of the time. I wondered what each one was thinking. I would try to find out later.

After dinner, Father and Joseph went down into the basement to the completely equipped work room with, among other equipment, a fly-tying workbench. Father had made a seventy-four drawer cabinet to hold all his hooks, leaders, tinsel, silk, feathers and vises for manufacturing trout and bass flies.

Joseph was most admiring of the deft way Father handled this delicate process. As I came down the stairs after helping with the dishes, I heard, much to my surprise, Father inviting Joseph to visit us in the Northwoods. This was unique.

Father had warned me, "Do not invite anyone to visit the Lone Larch cottage. You will be inundated with company who will bring a ham and expect to stay a week."

He need not have worried because Joseph hated being a house guest so did not accept the rare invitation.

ON MY OWN

I started practicing medicine that Fall at University Hospital, a small private institution owned by Dr. Charles Daniels, one of Father's close friends.

He gave me the use of a tiny office in the basement where several other members of the staff were located. I was grateful, first, because it cut office rent out of my overhead and, second, because my cubicle was next to Dr. Irish's office, one of my Pediatric professors. I had always admired this handsome man with his curly white hair and bright blue eyes.

He had a wry sense of humor and, between patients, we had many a laugh over his stories. One which was particularly typical of him was about a brash new intern who came up to Dr. Irish while he was making rounds.

He held out his hand and said, "I don't think you know me, but I'm your new intern."

Dr. Irish held out his hand and said, "I'm Irish."

The intern looked a bit blank for a minute, then took his hand and replied, "Oh, is that so? I'm Jewish."

Dr. Irish smiled his thin smile and answered, "Don't guild the lily."

This was particularly funny to me because the intern, Herman Goldsmith, had been in my section all through medical school and I had never seen him taken aback before.

Dr. Irish showed me many interesting cases during the year

and I was impressed with the thoroughness of his examinations. He would look, feel and listen carefully but gently and, when he was finished, he would hand the child a lollipop and dismiss him or her with a pat on the shoulder and say. "That's all!" The children would leave happy.

I thought, maybe their mothers and dentists would not have approved of this bribe, but the children did. They were never reluctant to go into his examining room and knew just where he kept the sweets.

Dr. Irish was a formidable teacher and so was Dr. Davidson. The intern and resident staff were terrified of the head of the hospital so I was glad I had taken internship and residency elsewhere.

The Head of the Department of OB and Gyne was Dr. Roger Burns, a stern, officious man who had insisted that his only son, Carl, study medicine. That young man was much more interested in the interior of cars than he was in the insides of people. He was a great trial to his father and also to Dr. Davidson because of his antics during his internship. If he had been anyone else's son, his internship would have been terminated promptly. But since his father was so influential, Dr. Davidson tried to ignore his capers.

One day, I was just leaving the hospital when I met Dr. Davidson and his entourage of house staff and attending men. The loudspeaker called out, "Dr. Carl Burns, come to the front lobby immediately. Dr. Carl Burns, please report to the lobby."

There was a flurry of upturned faces including that of Dr. Davidson as a white uniformed figure slid quickly down the banister and landed on his seat at Dr. Davidson's feet.

Dr. Davidson was purple and speechless, but not young Dr. Carl Burns, who got up, dusted himself off and remarked, "She did say immediately, didn't she?"

It became a watch word at the hospital.

I hadn't been seeing Joseph as much since the Fair closed and the Globe Players returned to England. I missed our intellectually stimulating evenings together. I wondered whether it was Shakespeare, or myself, which made him so attentive.

My practice was growing slowly, with most of my patients coming from Oak Park. Word spread among my high school and college classmates that I had hung up my shingle. Soon, I was looking around for additional office space in Oak Park. A physician father of one of my classmates was willing to give me space four days a week for a very small rental, so all I needed was a car.

I approached Father blithely about it. It probably was an inopportune time, because he was at his workbench in the basement writing checks for a multitude of bills.

"Now that I have both Oak Park and Chicago offices, I must have a car. How much can we afford?"

Father turned halfway toward me on his stool, "Where do you get this *must* and *we* business? I have sent you through eight years of college and medical school and three years of internship and residency and that's that! You are now on your own."

I was amazed. All my life I had been supported and suddenly the bottom had dropped out of my finances. If I had realized what a small salary Father had been receiving all those years, I would have been surprised that he could have managed at all.

"But what can I do? I don't have any money to buy a car!" My voice was plaintive — a tune that sometimes moved Father. This time it did not work.

"You'll think of something, but let me out of it."

I ran upstairs to Mother who was placidly working on a quilt.

"What can I do? Father won't buy me a car and I need it now that I have two offices."

She looked at me speculatively. "Do you have any friends who would lend you the money? How much does a small car cost?"

"I priced a Model T Ford yesterday and it was five hundred dollars brand new. The Ford dealer gave me a reduced price on it because he knew Father.   His place is near the medical school."

"I'm sure you'll find someone who will help you," Mother said calmly, returning to her quilting.   I knew she would have given me the money if she had it, but Father controlled the finances as he did everything else in the family.   These Pennsylvania Dutchmen!

Then a wave of remorse engulfed me. I really was ungrateful. I had been so used to receiving most anything I needed that I was programmed to believe it was my due.   Everyone said all only children were spoiled and I guess they were right.   I went up to my room and spent the rest of the afternoon being depressed and hating myself.

The next day, while making rounds on the two patients I had at the University Hospital, the Head Nurse noticed my unhappy expression.   "Where's our smiling woman doctor?" she asked.

At least she did not say *hen-medic!* I thought.

Miss Boardman invited me into her little office and offered me a cup of tea.   She was from England and thought this was a panacea for practically everything.   After a few sips of this British penicillin, I told Miss B my troubles.

"Why, is that all that's bothering you?" said Miss Boardman. "That is easily remedied." She took her check book out of her purse.

I couldn't believe my luck.

"But you hardly know me.   How fast do you think I can pay you back?"

Miss Boardman answered, "I'm not worried.   I see how conscientious you are about your patients, how you stay up with them all night if you are worried about them.   I know you will have a good-sized practice in no time."

I was so surprised and touched by this unexpected trust that my eyes filled with tears as I accepted the five hundred dollar check.

"I'll pay you back as soon as I'm able.   Would you like an

IOU?"

She shook her head. "That won't be necessary. I'm putting more than money on the line."

I never forgot the little Londoner who raised my depressed mood to one of thankfulness and elation.

I couldn't wait to drive my new car home to show my family. I remembered the long hours of driving, backing and parking when my father first taught me to drive.

He'd said, "Before you drive alone, every move must be just a reflex. You must not think before you act. It would take too much time." So for months on weekends we drove out to an area in River Forest where the streets were paved but no houses had been built.

I learned to back the car, do U turns, signal and park parallel to the right curb and to the left curb. All my life, I would be grateful for the intensive rigorous training I had received.

So, that glorious day when I took the whole family for a ride, I demonstrated the skills which my determined father had taught me.

The family had fun in my shiny, new, Black Ford and it reminded me of riding in Grandfather's Packard when I was seventeen and back in Pennsylvania. It had been the first automobile in the little town of Red Hill and had caused a lot of commotion with the people and the animals. The large limousine had a folding top with isinglass curtains which pulled down to keep the rain out, not that they did much good. The thing I had liked most was the Klaxon horn and the buggy whip, used to keep horses from getting to close. What an innocent age it had been.

But this car was different. It was my very own, that is, after I paid off the loan from Miss Boardman. I had a warm, grateful feeling whenever I turned on the ignition of the Model T. I paid her back at one hundred dollars a month plus a bonus gift — a lovely, hand knit, white wool sweater that Miss B could wear to work.

When I gave her the last check Miss Boardman smiled, gave me a hug and said, "I knew you could do it."

The two offices were moderately busy. I liked the clientele of my Oak Park office better because many of the parents were former classmates. Some of the patients at the Chicago office had been former patients at Cook County Children's Hospital and I felt guilty charging their parents even a small fee.

One day, a disreputable looking man asked the receptionist if he might talk to me. She agreed, but wondered when she recognized him, whether it had been wise. He had a wild expression in his eyes and he looked as though he had been crying.

"I don't know whether you remember me or not. My son was Harry McPherson. He was a patient of yours in the TB ward."

I remembered Harry very well. He had been an undernourished tow-headed darling with a disseminated tuberculosis so far advanced that his lungs looked like a snowstorm on X-ray. His father had refused to believe the diagnosis and had taken the boy home after signing a release about a year ago.

He had taken the boy to various doctors until he found one who told him his son would recover and that there was nothing wrong with him.

I was horrified at such poor medical judgment. Mr. McPherson became more excited as he continued with his story.

Suddenly he pulled out a .32 caliber revolver and laid it on my desk.

"Tell me, doctor. If I had listened to you and left Harry in the hospital, would he be alive today?"

I looked into the man's troubled eyes. I felt the horrible weight of guilt weighing on his soul.

"Mr. McPherson, I honestly do not believe anything you could have done would have saved him. It was such an advanced tuberculosis that the germs were in his blood stream. We have no medicine to cure that."

Mr. McPherson laid his head on my desk and cried bitterly. I patted his arm.

Finally he raised his head, wiped his eyes and with a great sigh, picked up the gun and put it in his jacket.

"You know, doctor, if you had said you could have saved him, I would have shot myself right then."

I ushered him out quietly and after he had left, I went into Dr. Irish's office and told him the whole story. I was weak. "When I saw the gun I really thought he was going to kill me."

Dr. Irish laughed, "I guess your time has not come yet. You have too many young lives to save!"

But somehow this experience took the bloom off the Chicago office. I was seeing more patients in Oak Park so decided to concentrate on working there.

Joseph called me up one day, "Is this my ex-resident?"

I immediately knew who it was. I'd have known that beautifully modulated voice anywhere.

"Yes, it is. What a pleasant surprise! How are you, Joseph?"

"I'm fine but I just fired my associate."

"Why? He seemed like such a pleasant young man."

"That's the trouble. He was too pleasant, especially with the student nurses in the linen closet."

"Oh?" I hoped he was going to ask me an important question, and he did.

"Would you like to be my new associate?"

"How would Dr. Blatt like that? He prides himself on never having had a woman associate!"

"I've already asked him if I could appoint you."

"Oh you did, did you? How did you know I'd say yes?"

I could hear him chuckle. "I kind of thought you would."

"Well, Joseph, you were right. I would consider it an honor to be your associate. I really enjoy working with you."

"The feeling is mutual. I'll see you tonight at the staff meeting."

The attending men and other associates were very friendly that evening. They acted as though they had not seen me for years, although it had only been six months.

Dr. Blatt rapped for order.

He said, "Before we read the minutes of the previous meeting, I'd like to introduce our newest associate, Dr. Dorothy Welker. She will work with Dr. Joseph Greengard."

After much clapping and one muted "Hurrah," Dr. Blatt continued, "She was a satisfactory resident and I am sure she will be a satisfactory associate as well. She can now carry Dr. Greengard's bag."

I blushed as I remembered how angry I had been to have to carry Dr. Blatt's bag — just like a bearer on safari, I used to think. Nevertheless, I stood up and made a polite little comment about how happy I was to be a member of the staff and I really was.

MEETING MRS. GREENGARD

Working with Joseph was pure pleasure because he was such an excellent pediatrician. He had a great store of medical knowledge and could express himself well when writing on the charts. In fact, we used to write little notes to one another.

One time, we were both greatly concerned over a black boy on the TB ward who had both tuberculosis and sickle cell anemia.

I wrote, "At 10:00 a.m. today T.J. had a severe hemoptysis."

The next day Dr. Greengard wrote, "Don't scare me like that! I think you meant epistaxis."

The following day I answered, "I am sorry! You would think by now I would know the difference between a hemorrhage from the lung and a nosebleed! Are you going to get a new and smarter associate?"

Dr. Greengard wrote, "Not yet, but be careful. I don't want to have a heart attack."

So the months went on. I made rounds in the mornings at County and saw patients in my Oak Park office in the afternoons. Joseph would take me to a play or concert weekends and gradually we became more involved emotionally.

One day Joseph asked me to marry him. I had been afraid that was coming so I had my answer ready. "I am very fond of you, Joseph, but I don't think I am quite ready for marriage.

Sometime ago, I was badly hurt by falling in love with the wrong person, and I don't want that to happen again."

He looked as though he had been slapped across the face. For many years, he had been running away from pursuing females and now here I was reversing the process.

He drove me home without saying another word and a few days later he left for a month's Caribbean cruise.

Two parcels arrived soon after that: an album of Gilbert and Sullivan's *Mikado*, which we both had enjoyed in concert, and a huge florist box of eighteen, deep red roses with dozens of large white gardenias scattered over the surface.

A card lay on top saying, simply, "I'm sorry."

I was floored. Nothing like that had ever happened to me. In addition, every day an exquisitely worded letter arrived describing the sights of the cruise. Not a word, though, about his disappointment or about love.

I talked the whole thing over with my parents. I had promised my mother not to get married until I had an established medical practice. I fulfilled the promise, so that was no obstacle.

Joseph was a Jew, but this was no obstacle as far as my parents and I were concerned. They liked him a lot and respected him for his brilliant mind and the success he had made in medical writings.

I became more fond of him as time went on. Absence makes the heart grow fonder, I thought – and not *for somebody else!* as the old joke went.

When Joseph returned we had a wonderful reunion. We were parked out at Montrose Harbor because we both loved looking at the Lake with the lights reflected on it. All at once, Joseph took me in his arms and gave me a long tender kiss. In the midst of this, a gruff policeman's voice said, "Come up for air!"

He had turned his flashlight on our faces as we startled apart. Whereupon he gave us a lecture about the dangers of being attacked at night on the Chicago Lakefront.

I was terribly embarrassed.

Of course, he had only been doing his duty, but he need not have done it in such a crude way! I cried all the way home and what was worse, I felt Joseph was angry. I did not know whether he was annoyed with me, or with that creep of a policeman – or with himself for getting me in that uncomfortable situation. Anyhow, he said a cool goodnight when he deposited me on my Oak Park door step.

About this time, Joseph's mother had a coronary thrombosis. Joseph had lived with his mother for several years after his father had died. When Mrs. Greengard had recovered from her heart attack enough to go to her daughter's apartment, Joseph found a small flat of his own on Sheridan Road and invited me to meet his uncle there. I volunteered to make dinner for the three of us and since I did not know anything about cooking, decided that a steak would be easiest.

I had V8 to start with, the steak and baked potatoes, frozen peas, rolls, and ice cream for dessert. It was as simple a dinner as I could make.

Joseph's uncle, who was the youngest of Mrs. Greengard's family of four brothers and four sisters, was only ten years older than Joseph. He was a wizened little architect who loved Joseph dearly since he had no children of his own. As a matter of fact, six of the family were single and lived together in a huge apartment on Junior Terrace. They all admired and respected Joseph intensely and were interested in this *woman doctor* friend.

So I was nervous about meeting Bernhard and, especially, cooking my first meal for him and Joseph. I knew he would have lots of things to tell the family when he went home. I borrowed Joseph's key and shopped for the ingredients for our meal and went up to his flat to see where the dishes and utensils were kept.

It was a small studio apartment with a nice view of the lake, but a totally inadequate kitchen.

I did the best I could, under the circumstances, but the dinner was only mediocre. The steaks came out medium instead of medium rare the way Joseph and I liked ours. The rolls were a little dried out and the ice cream too soft.

Nevertheless Bernhard said he admired my cooking; especially the steak which was "just right," according to him.

We liked each other immediately, because our artistic tastes were similar. The impressionist painters were our favorites. In music, we preferred Bach, Brahms, Schumann, Chopin and Mozart, and we'd both enjoyed reading the Forsyte Saga.

Joseph was very quiet, just sitting back enjoying our easy rapport.

When Bernhard left, he took Joseph to one side and whispered something to him. Joseph later told me that he'd said, "I am favorably impressed with your friend. I was afraid she would have bleached blonde hair."

Joseph laughed at Bernhard's naiveté. He must have thought that all non-Jewish girls were scheming hussies with heavy makeup.

Mrs. Greengard's health had continued to improve but since she was prejudiced against anyone, especially a Gentile, who had "designs" on her son, Joseph was afraid to bring me around to meet her.

I'd been waiting for Joseph to propose again, but since he didn't I decided he was afraid of being turned down a second time.

After the happy evening with Bernhard, I decided to take the initiative. We were sitting in the dark in Joseph's apartment looking at Lake Michigan with the streams of gold headlights driving south and the red tail lights going north.

Boats were bobbing in the harbor and some of them were lit up with reflections from their lights casting streamers over the waves.

"Isn't this peaceful and lovely?" I said, giving Joseph's warm comfortable hand a little squeeze.

He smiled and said, "It is so pleasant here, I hate to take you home."

This was my chance. I said, "Maybe someday you won't have to."

"Are you sure?" he asked. "I don't want to be refused again!"

"I am sure, "I said, "I was so impressed with all your letters from the Caribbean. I was really angry at myself for having been so negative."

Joseph gave me a big hug and in his arms I felt safer than I ever had. "Oh, Joseph let's get married soon," I said.

The next free day we went to Peacock's and picked out a perfect blue-white, half karat diamond to be set with three small stones on each side of it and a platinum wedding ring to match with eighteen chips set in groups of three. Joseph apologized for the size of the stone, but I would rather have a flawless blue-white diamond than a larger imperfect one.

A month later, we were having lunch at the Mill Run Inn, a charming spot on the Fox River. Joseph reached in his pocket and brought out a small velvet box with the rings in them.

My heart gave a little flip-flop of delight. They looked so perfect, so handsome, just like Joseph. There was a quality of integrity about the rings that reminded me of him. It was most appealing. He slipped the engagement ring on the third finger of my left hand, but did not kiss me in such a public place. That could wait for later.

After that, when I was percussing a patient and saw the diamond shining on my left hand, I took special care with diagnosing the sounds because I was reminded Joseph always was so thorough with his diagnosis. I had a great deal to live up to as his associate and his wife.

Joseph and I were married May 10, 1935 in Harvey, Illinois. His mother was still bedridden and etiquette in those days meant a quiet wedding out of respect for her condition so we did not tell anyone – but as we went out the door, my mother said to Joseph, "Be kind to her." She knew.

We were married by a Justice of Peace, Joseph McCarthy, a big, hearty man who read a long ceremony and quoted from the Bible. His secretary and a one-armed woman served as our witnesses and admired my lovely gardenia corsage from Joseph.

Then Joseph McCarthy gave us our marriage license. It was an elaborately decorated, 20 by 24 inch parchment with the bridal couple seated in a gondola guided by a fat little cupid wearing a derby. We both loved that cupid.

The honeymoon was short — a weekend in Brown County, Indiana. It was an artists' colony where we purchased a tea set of green and tan native pottery, our first household possession. This was in the midst of the depression, so even a small item was a big investment. I treasured it all my life, even more than the elegant wedding presents which we received later.

Joseph's apartment was our first home, but it really was not very satisfactory because our marriage had to be so secret. I'd been staying at my parents' home nights and we didn't like that arrangement, but we knew it was only temporary. Of course, Mother and Father knew by this time, but we thought nobody else did. Then one day I overheard Grandmother say to Mother, "They are married, I can tell."

My mother laughed, "How can you tell?"

"Oh, by their expressions. They look like two cats that have finished a saucer of cream!"

But the big hurdle for me was being introduced to Joseph's mother. She was a formidable woman, the matriarch of the clan. Everyone, except Joseph, was a little afraid of her and carried out her every wish. In addition, now that she had suffered a heart attack, they did not want to precipitate another one by crossing her.

We spent long hours discussing how to solve this delicate problem. We decided that we would set the supposed date of the wedding for July thirteenth — a lucky number since Joseph had been born on the thirteenth and we had become engaged on the thirteenth.

We would go to Joseph's sister, Dotto's, apartment and tell his mother that we were getting married that day, thus squelching, we hoped, any discussion about a formal wedding.

I did not sleep well the night before, worrying as to what would happen. Joseph had told me how outspoken his mother was. He said, "She prides herself on saying just what she thinks, no matter how it offends."

"I like that," I had answered. "I hate deceitful people, but I do hope she will approve of me."

Joseph smiled, "Well I do and that is all that matters."

I wished I could be calm as Joseph seemed to be as we walked up the stairs to Dotto and Leo's second floor apartment where my mother-in-law was staying. I felt much better when I was ushered in by a charming, sweet-faced woman who was a few years younger than Joseph. She greeted us warmly and led the way to a rear bedroom.

Mother Greengard was propped up in bed with a hand knit shawl over her shoulders. She had a heavy head of grey-white hair in two braids and an aristocratic profile.

My heart skipped a beat. I sat down on a chair by the bed. What was going to happen now? Joseph's sister had told her that we were engaged, so at least she knew that much.

"This is Joseph's fiancée," said Dotto.

"I've been so anxious to meet you," I said, "but we did not want to disturb you until you felt better."

Mrs. Greengard smiled, "I am much better now. They even allow me to get up and walk around a little, but I am very unsteady on my feet."

"I know how that is because I was off my feet for quite a while a few years ago."

Mrs. Greengard looked worried. "Was it anything serious? I hope you are all right now."

"Oh, I'm fine. I guess I was just exhausted from working too hard as an intern." I immediately thought that I'd said the wrong thing. Joseph's mother would worry that Joseph was getting a fragile wife.

Joseph must have read my thought because he said, "I'll say Dorothy is fine. She makes rounds at County and wears me out!"

We all laughed. Dotto said, "Joseph told us you are on your way to get married. He will have to get you a nice corsage."

I blushed. I hated to deceive these friendly people, so I said, "Joseph has given me enough flowers to last me the rest of my life. He knows how to woo a girl."

It was Joseph's turn to look embarrassed. In order to cover his confusion, he looked at his watch and said, "Well, I guess it is time to go."

I sighed, "I hate to leave when I have just met you, Mrs. Greengard, but I don't want to tire you out."

She held out her hand and took mine in both of hers, "Take good care of my 'schatsero'. Do you know what that means?"

My eyes smiled into her loving ones. "Yes I do. It means 'little sweetheart'!" I silently thanked Charlie for his lessons in Yiddish and German.

Joseph's mother was pleased. Here was a girl she could relate to. Years later, when I confided my doubts and fears of meeting her, she said, "As soon as I looked at you, I knew everything would be all right because I could see you loved my Joseph."

What a large leap that had been over the huge crevasse of prejudice.

As Joseph drove back to the apartment he said, "I have to give you credit. You handled that situation just right. I've never seen Mother so friendly to a stranger before. She is usually very much on guard."

"I'm so glad," I said with a sigh of relief, letting my armor down.

DOCTOR, WIFE, MOTHER

We started looking for a larger apartment. That was quite a chore since we needed a living room with an unbroken wall long enough to accommodate a large walnut bookcase the Uncle Bernhard designed for us. Besides this, we wanted to be near the Lake and yet have a reasonable rental.

Joseph had just started out practicing on his own. He'd left his association with Dr. Blatt which made me happy. I still resented that stiff necked tyrant and, recently, Joseph had grown tired of his dictatorial ways too.

Finally, after many discouraging searches, we found what we wanted on the eighth floor of a building near Joseph's office. It was not on the lake but, the cost of lakefront apartments was prohibitive on our small income and, if I stood on tiptoes looking out of the bedroom window, I could catch a glimpse of a small strip of blue between buildings. It would have to do.

The place was called "The Hazel Crest" and it was just across the street from a public garage where we could keep our cars. It had an elevator and no long corridors which always made me think of jails.

Joseph was working very hard. I had been appointed attending *man* at Grant Hospital in return for which I manned the free Baby Clinic for indigent families. This met one morning a week and was under the fierce direction of Mrs. Jones, a most efficient nurse. She was director of all the nurses in the outpatient clinics and bossed the doctors unmercifully. Because she was just as severe with her own staff and very kind to the patients, the doctors did not resent it. As a matter of fact, they all liked her and, what is more important, respected her.

I was frightened the first day as I dressed in a white gown for the Clinic, but Mrs. Jones put me at ease.

"It will be difficult for you to fill Dr. Barnes' shoes. He was here for fifteen years and is an excellent pediatrician. He is now sitting under his citrus trees, enjoying the cool breezes of Florida.

"But I am sure you will catch on quickly. We have some fine volunteers who will take dictation as you examine the patients and give the mothers directions. If any of the infants need to be hospitalized you may admit them on your own service."

Instead of the student nurses that usually helped with the Clinic, Mrs. Jones attended my early sessions. I didn't know this was unusual. Mrs. Jones had many important administrative chores, but whether or not it was from curiosity, because I was the first woman doctor to be given this post, she was a constant observer at the two to three hour Clinic.

It made it a great deal easier for me and after a few sessions of 20 to 25 patients, the clinic functioned smoothly. The team of Dr. Welker, Mrs. Jones and two volunteers was a pleasure to watch. Or so it seemed as there was always an intern or two hanging around. Soon I found myself teaching them.

My enthusiasm for the clinic bubbled over at home. "What are you so pleased about?" asked my new husband.

"I never knew running a baby clinic could be such fun. Mrs. Jones is terrific. There are no tiresome delays the way there were at County Outpatients. She has each baby undressed, weighed and measured by the time I'm finished with the previous one, and the volunteers really know their stuff. They take dictation like pros."

He smiled. "You are so young and refreshing. I know many

doctors who would be bored stiff with that job."

"Oh, how could they be? I just love examining the little bunnies. They are so soft and cuddly. I do hate it when they are terribly sick, though. It frightens me."

And there was a good reason to be frightened. Without antibiotics and good intravenous therapy, infant mortality in the 1930's was staggering. Many times, the best we could do was to give them oxygen. It was heart breaking to watch them struggle for breath.

I was particularly fond of the prematures, so transparent, tiny and vulnerable. So when I was asked two years later whether or not I would like to establish the first Premature Station on the North Side, I gladly accepted.

I had taken care of many prematures at County and with the experience of doing autopsies on prematures in pathology, I felt I knew something about them.

"Do you really think I can do it?" I asked.

Joseph encouraged me. "Of course you can. Read everything you can find in the medical literature on the subject, get the hospital board to buy you the proper equipment, have good registered nurses and trained interns and you'll be all right."

I looked at him gratefully. When I needed support, he was always there.

"Thank you, darling. With your advice, I guess I can make it!"

I ordered thirteen Isolettes at one thousand dollars a piece; the first ones used in the Midwest. It was a gamble, but I had been impressed with the results I'd seen at a post graduate course on prematures at Cornell. The Isolettes controlled humidity, temperature and oxygen concentration.

Now my schedule was really heavy. Hospital rounds at County *and* Grant, the Premature Station and the free Baby Clinic filled my mornings. Afternoon appointments at my Oak Park office kept me running all day long.

Joseph was a full professor at the University of Illinois

Medical School; plus attending man at County, Sara Morris Hospital at Michael Reese. He also was working very hard making five to ten house calls a day

Eventually, I had to give up my beloved Oak Park office. Joseph and I had several long discussions about it. A very attractive suite had opened up on Broadway and Lawrence. It had a large reception room, a receptionist's office, laboratory, four examining rooms, and a fluoroscopic room (if we could afford a fluoroscope).

In order to rent the space, we had to give up our other offices. Joseph didn't mind at all, since he was just subletting, but I hated leaving my old hometown, even though I didn't live there anymore. At least four times a week, I had to admit it was difficult making house calls there. The North Side of Chicago, where we lived, was twelve miles away and, often, I would no sooner get home than I would have to turn around and drive back. Besides that, the night calls were impossible.

So, reluctantly, I severed my connection with Oak Park and outfitted the office on the North Side of Chicago. Some of my patients followed me there, but many transferred to other pediatricians closer to Oak Park. I couldn't blame them, but I did miss them.

At first Joseph and I shared the same afternoons at the office, but as our practices increased in numbers, we found it less confusing to have alternate afternoons. We tried several nurses without success until a tall, young, registered nurse applied for the double job of nurse-receptionist. She was pretty and had a pleasant smile, but also a firm manner as though she was saying to the children, "Behave yourself and do what the doctor asks or you'll get into trouble."

This nurse, Kay Gilman, stayed with us as long as we had the office. She was a true find, managing both the office and us in a most respectful, unobtrusive manner. We were very fond of her.

It was exciting fitting out the office. I always liked interior design and made long, blue and white, lined drapes for all the windows. The office was located on the prow of the seventh floor of the huge bank building. One set of windows faced North and the rest East, with a fantastic view of the city. A side benefit, at dusk, was watching the traffic slowly light up along the street. Joseph and I always did that when we had a break between patients, which was very seldom. It was our only recreation.

One of Joseph's cousins painted murals on the walls of the third examining room depicting brightly colored circus performers, clowns, bareback riders and a musician tooting a strange horn. The children loved them and so did I. We had a tank of tropical fish set in the reception room wall. It was a great trial to Kay. Every day, she had to clean the children's hand prints from the glass, because they always stood, spellbound, leaning on the glass, fish gazing. At least it kept them occupied while they waited.

I was exhausted, so tired that it was hard for me to cook dinner at night. Eating out took too much time and money, so we hired a woman to make the evening meal for us. In spite of that, I continued to be nauseated every evening. I went to Joseph's friend and classmate, Dr. Heath, an internist.

He called it nervous exhaustion and advised me to take some time off. I hated it and became restless wandering around the apartment, but my symptoms did not go away. Finally, I followed Joseph's advice and went to my parents' house for a few days. I wasn't there very long before Grandmother came up with a diagnosis.

"I think you are pregnant," she said confidently.

"How can I be? I'm still menstruating."

"That doesn't matter, " said Nanny, "I've known lots of girls who did that the first month or two."

"But Dr. Heath said it was nervous exhaustion and he's supposed to be an excellent doctor."

"Nervous exhaustion my foot! Have you never heard of morning sickness? Well, this is evening sickness. You just have your time table reversed. Go get a rabbit test."

I felt better already. I had always thought Nanny missed her calling. With her large build, confident manner and ability to offer comfort, she'd have made an excellent physician, but nobody heard of woman doctors when she was a girl. That's why she was so happy to see my success as a doctor.

Nanny's lay diagnosis was correct and Joseph and I were delighted about it. Now that I knew all was well, I went back to work and, after a month or two more, I could eat dinner again.

So, with the prospect of an increased family we went apartment hunting again. This time, we were better off financially with two practices booming, very low income tax rates and no such thing as medical malpractice insurance – nobody thought of suing doctors in those days.

We found an apartment in a good neighborhood about two blocks from the lake. It had a sun porch in front with a large bay window, a good sized living room with one long, unbroken wall, two bedrooms and baths, a dining room and kitchen, plus a maid's room, bath and back porch. My only reservation was that it was on the third floor and had a long hall.

I shook that off as unimportant when I thought of my poor mother, living in a fifth floor apartment in New York City when my father had been working on his Ph.D. at Columbia. Mother was afraid to leave my large wicker buggy in the lobby, so she hauled it, with me inside, up four flights of stairs, ending up so breathless she almost fainted.

Years later, I teased her saying, "You should have left me downstairs. I'm sure the buggy was more valuable."

Since I was considered *an elderly primipara* at thirty-two, Joseph thought I should have a top-flight obstetrician. Father suggested Dr. Falls, the Head of the O.B. Department at the University of Illinois Medical School.

I knew him socially when he used to come to my folk's house and play Ragtime on the piano when I was a little girl.

After he had examined me, he looked very grave, "I hope

your husband does not have a large frame?" he questioned me.

"Oh, you know him," I answered, "Dr. Joseph Greengard, from Pediatrics."

"Oh, yes, I remember Joseph. A very good teacher and only about five feet eight or nine inches tall." he said approvingly.

"What are you worried about?"

"Well, Dorothy, you have a justo-minor pelvis, which as you know, does not leave much room for the baby to pass through. The smaller the husband, likewise the baby, and better off for both mother and baby. We can always do a Caesarian, but I hope we won't have to."

I gave a little shudder. In those days Caesarians were only done as a last resort with sometimes disastrous results to both the mother and child.

The rest of the pregnancy went along uneventfully, with me working until two days before the baby was due. I was sleeping peacefully at about two a.m. when, suddenly, I dreamt I was drowning. I woke up with a cry which frightened Joseph. We both realized the bag of waters had ruptured prematurely.

He helped me out of bed and replaced the mattress pad and bed clothes. We waited expectantly for the labor pains to start. Nothing happened, so we tried to go back to sleep without much success. The night seemed endless.

We called Dr. Falls at seven o'clock in the morning and arranged to meet him at Grant Hospital. He examined me and told me to go home and call when the labor pains began. They started about a week later with a bang.

Joseph drove me to the hospital and then a painful, 24 hour labor began. The fact that the bag of waters had ruptured so long before, kept the flushing out of the baby from happening which would have made the delivery easier.

Dr. Falls offered me a shot of morphine to ease the pain but I refused it. I had seen too many babies die because of pain killers given to the mothers.

The pain was excruciating. Joseph never left me except to

get a little food and the nurse took the opportunity to give me a lecture about not minding the pain.

Joseph came in at the tail end of the diatribe and really was disgusted with the nurse.

"I bet she never had a baby or she would not be so heartless," he said, but, typical to his character, he did not bawl her out. I never heard him scold anyone.

Finally, Dr. Falls came in for the fourth time that day. He shook his head. "Your uterus is forming a Bandle's Ring which is a localized muscular contraction. Your cervix is not dilating and that is why the labor is not progressing."

Joseph and I knew this was serious because Bandle's Ring was a dangerous sign that the uterus might rupture. So I had to take a morphine shot after all. The pains stopped temporarily.

Dr. Falls did not go home after that, but kept listening to the baby's heart beat. If it had become too fast or too slow he would have done an emergency Caesarian operation. Fortunately the little fetus cooperated and her heart kept up a steady firm beat.

After my rest, Dr. Falls told me that my cervix was dilating at last and in another hour, on November 3, 1937, our baby arrived. She was a beautiful infant in spite of a black eye and a broken collar bone, the result of the long dry labor.

Joseph went home after I was brought back to the room and as he left with his shoulders bent forward and his steps slow, I felt so sorry for him that I made up my mind I would not put him through that trauma again. Watching someone you love suffer is ten times as difficult as going through it yourself.

I was floating on a cloud. Whether it was due to the morphine shot or the wonderful relief of not having any more pain, I didn't know, but all my life I remembered the euphoria of the rest of that night. I just lay there, looking out at the sky line with three tall spires visible from my window. I felt they had a religious significance and I thanked God for the miracle of birth and for my lovely little girl.

HEARTH AND HOME

After the usual week's stay in the hospital, the homecoming was glorious. Joseph carried Joanne into her nursery and introduced her to Mary, our maid. Mary was a young Irish immigrant we'd hired to take care of the apartment and the meals, but I did not want to have a nurse for the baby. I took a leave of absence so I could devote all my time to taking care of this precious gift. I felt I could learn more practical pediatrics this way than from all the textbooks and lectures I had read.

It was not that easy, because I could not nurse Joanne. After all the encouragement I had given my new mothers, it was a great disappointment that I was unable to, but when I had gone in for my first prenatal examination, Dr. Falls had shaken his head sadly as he looked at my breasts, "You're no good," he'd said.

"Why?"

"Because you have inverted nipples. You can massage them and try to pull them out, but I doubt if it will do any good. There's nothing there for the baby to latch on to."

I was disgusted. I knew all the advantages of breast milk — which carried antibodies from the mother's previous infections to the baby. Thus the infant was not nearly so prone to get upper respiratory infections, whooping cough or chicken pox as long as she had breast milk. In addition the curd tension of breast milk was much lower, and the calcium content and protein were different than cow's milk. After all, the needs of a large boned calf were entirely different than those of a seven pound baby.

Besides — and this was most important of all — breast milk was sterile, which cut down on the number of gastrointestinal infections, such as diarrhea, which the baby might have. Knowing all these reasons, I was especially interested in getting my breast milk to the baby. I rented an electric breast pump and tried desperately to get even one feeding a day of breast milk for Joanne, but no luck. The more I tried, the more tense I became, and the less breast milk I manufactured.

"Oh, why am I not a stoic person?" I asked Joseph.

"Let's face it Dorothy," he said, "You're just not a good cow!"

So Joanne became a colicky baby and cried bitterly all through the dinner hour from six to eight. I tried changing her diapers, trying to make her comfortable in a different position, giving her sips of brandy and warm water, but the only thing that would help was to pick her up, walk her or jiggle the bassinet, all *no-nos*.

Joanne enjoyed all the attention and soon learned the way to get it was to bellow loudly and get blue in the face. With my soft-hearted nature, I could not stand to see her "suffer", so Joseph and I took turns eating our dinners alone while the other one entertained Joanne.

At least we knew colic did not last forever; three months was the most one could expect it to endure and, sure enough, Joanne became docile at that time.

I gradually went back to my medical duties, first the free Baby Clinic then the Premature Station. Mary loved taking the baby for walks over to a nearby park, so we hired another maid, a friend of Mary's from Ireland, to help with the household chores. I returned to my office hours, but felt cheated whenever I thought of Joanne being cared for by Mary. I did not realize how attached Mary had become to her until one terrible night when Joanne had a high temperature and the croup. I looked up

and saw Mary standing in the doorway of the nursery.
I could not believe the hostile look on her face. She brushed
past me and tried to take Joanne out of my arms.

"Give her to me!" she shouted. "You don't know how to take
care of her, she's mine."

I called Joseph and he quickly insisted that Mary go back to
her room. Both Joseph and I were shocked at the intensity of her
emotions. The next morning I arranged for Mary to see a
psychiatrist. She refused.

"Then I am afraid you will have to leave," I told her. "If,
however, you see Dr. Evans as I have arranged, and he says it is
all right for you to continue to work here, I will take you back.
That's fair isn't it?"

Mary nodded reluctantly and I called a taxi to take her to the
Doctor's office, which was nearby. In an hour the phone rang. It
was Dr. Evans.

"I am so glad you sent Mary to me," he said. "She is
seriously disturbed. I'm afraid she thinks your baby belongs to
her. Don't let her back into your house. She has homicidal
tendencies and is liable to kill you and kidnap your baby!"

I nearly dropped the phone. We'd never suspected Mary was
so unstable.

I felt sorry for her, but was terrified as well. I arranged for
her belongings to be gathered up by her friend, Elsie, and be
taken with a month's salary to a room several miles away. I
wrote Mary a note saying I would give her a satisfactory
reference if she applied to some family who did not have
children. I recommended that Mary go to a mental health clinic
as well.

Years later when I met Mary again. She was wheeling her
own infant in Lincoln park − a truly happy ending.

The apartment on Buena Avenue was roomy, but it had a
long hall which I detested. It was near the Lake and not too far
from Grant Hospital but to me an apartment was only an
apartment and a house was more like a home. I had been raised

in houses first in Chicago, then in Oak Park and I always felt like an alien in an apartment.

For two and a half years, I kept showing houses I liked to Joseph. He definitely was not interested in any of them. One was a gorgeous old home on the lakefront in Evanston. It had a well kept, lush, green lawn sloping down to a concrete break water at the lake's edge. I was fascinated by its large rooms and pretty garden.

Joseph objected because of the breakwater. "One bad storm and it will be torn to bits. It would take over ten thousand dollars to replace and if we extend ourselves with two mortgages on the place, we might lose it."

I was never practical in money matters so I dismissed Joseph's objection and kept staunchly naming all its good points. We had the first real battle of our married life.

"I don't see why you think that will happen," I argued. "It has been standing there for forty years. Why should a storm affect it now?"

Joseph usually gave in to my wishes if he saw I really wanted something, but he was adamant on this decision.

"No, no, no!" he kept saying.

I cried myself to sleep many a night over Number 170 Front Street, Evanston, but Joseph acted as though he did not hear me.

Time proved Joseph right. The winter of 1940 came with many severe storms on Lake Michigan. Huge waves coming from the East buffeted the lakefront and torrents of rain, hail and snow raised the level of the lake twenty feet, the highest it had ever been since Chicago was settled.

After the last storm Joseph drove me to Evanston's shore line to see the damage. There was complete chaos with enormous chunks of concrete piled up on the once-beautiful lawn of Number 170.

He did not say, "I told you so," but I had to admit he had been right as usual. It was maddening. I knew it was lucky we hadn't bought my dream home, but it was still a bitter pill to swallow. By that time, however, we were already settled in our first home.

Not long after Joseph's refusal to buy the house in Evanston, he came home as excited as I had ever seen him. He handed me a telephone number. "Call up this realtor," he said. "I just made a house call on the Gerstleys' on North Virginia Avenue and their neighbors have a house for sale. The address is 5480."

He didn't have to ask twice. The next weekend, we went to see the white frame house with green shutters. An architect had bought five lots on the corner of Virginia and Balmoral. They were heavily wooded with old oak trees, wild plum and maple. He had built a house with a colonial doorway and a small covered stoop.

I stepped into a large foyer, with a charming mahogany and white painted staircase leading to the second floor. The living room was fourteen feet wide and forty feet long. The dining room was also large, plus there was a breakfast nook and workable kitchen with butler's pantry. For the first time in my life, I wanted to cook. The master bedroom and bath were adjacent to a good-sized library with bare walls ready for our bookcase.

On the second floor, I found two huge bedrooms, a tiny narrow play room and a bath all under the eaves.

I tried not to act as thrilled as I felt because Joseph was talking terms with the realtor. The asking price was ridiculously low, since the owner had lost it in bankruptcy and the bank was anxious to unload it. However Joseph was offering five hundred dollars less than the bank wanted and he stuck to that.

"How stubborn a man can be!" I thought, holding my breath for fear we would lose it. At last, Joseph's offer was accepted and we allowed the people renting there to stay until Spring when our apartment lease on Buena Avenue was up.

We found out later this was a mistake, since the renters did not water the flowers or rake up the multitude of leaves which ruined the lawn.

Whenever I had time, I spent the interim measuring the rooms, the windows and the kitchen spaces. I drew many sketches and cut out paper furniture to the size of the furniture we owned or had to buy.

We went downtown and picked out a down-pillowed davenport on which both of us could lie down together and watch television. The customers at Wilson's Furniture Store were amused to see us lying supine, side by side, to see whether or not we would fit. We also tried bouncing on the beds to see if they were comfortable. Mr. Jump, who later had his own furniture store, helped us make our decision and also did a little bouncing himself.

My desire for decorating was satisfied in picking out a bright, cardinal studded wall paper for the dining room and a blown up sepia photograph of Jackson Hole in Estes Park for one whole wall in the library. That was a dramatic success. Many a time when I was tired from hospital rounds, office hours and house calls I would sit across the room and join the fisherman in the landscape while Joseph worked at his desk.

We hired a young man, named Peter Neidenback, to do the gardening. We were fortunate in getting him. He had just returned from an apprenticeship in California with his uncle, a trained horticulturist. Peter's real trade was printing but, with the depression still going on, he needed extra work and liked my job of landscaping.

Peter and I planned a rock garden and a waterfall sloping from the back patio. He dug an irregular shaped pit and lined it with concrete for a goldfish pond, surrounded by ferns. We planted a mountain ash shading the whole complex. It was a delightful place leading over to the wild plum orchard by irregular sandstone stepping stones.

We found that rocks for the pool and rock garden were very expensive so we drove thirty miles out to an old quarry and picked up some beautifully weathered, brown and tan specimens and loaded them into the trunk of my Buick. Unfortunately, when we reached home, I found that one of the car's shocks was damaged. We had been too enthusiastic in our rock gathering. But it had been worth it. We never could have found aged specimens such as these in the Chicago nurseries.

In the Fall, we planted a thousand hybrid tulips along the back fence and driveway. These bulbs were among the first shipped from Holland after the war and each one was as big as my fist. The dealer had told us they were the only ones not eaten by the Dutch when they were starving during the war.

When they bloomed they were breathtaking; all colors, stripes, even black blossoms. We planted huge gold and purple irises behind them and blue dwarf phlox in front. It made a lovely, fifty-foot border. People walking along the alley stopped and stared and in the Fall helped themselves to some of the iris bulbs, much to my disgust.

I'd ordered chocolate brown carpeting for the first floor of the house and when it finally arrived it was a sickly, reddish tan. I sent it back, wrathfully, knowing it would be another three months before the right carpet arrived. At least the furniture was perfect, including the cherry dining room set, with ladder-back chairs and hutch to match. Mother began making needle point seats for the whole set. This nearly completed our dream house.

When the carpets finally arrived and were put in place, Joseph and I gave a house warming party. We were all set to have a blazing fire in the marble fireplace at the end of the room, when we discovered the fireplace had no chimney. The one we had seen from the outside of the house was on the South side and the fireplace was on the East side. It had been moved when the chimney caught fire several years before, but the owners just put it there for show, not for use.

I was deeply disappointed since I felt fireplaces added to the coziness of a house turning it into a home. When we priced the cost of opening up the old chimney, lining it and punching out a hole in the south wall, we decided that the coziness was not worth it! Well, I wasn't so sure at first, but then I knew Joseph was always right when it came to finances.

We weren't in our new house more than three months before I recognized my symptoms of pregnancy. Dr. Falls had told me not to have any more children because of my justo-minor pelvis, but I decided to take a chance anyhow. I was anxious to have another child because I did not want Joanne to have as lonely a childhood as I had. I thought a three year interval between siblings would be about right.

When my due date arrived, my second child did not cooperate. A week went by and then another week and nothing happened.

Eventually, I had to stop practicing. One day my hip just gave out and I fell. I had to be picked up off the sidewalk in front of my office and carried to my car. As soon as I was sitting down I was all right.

That evening there were radio and TV warnings of a severe snowstorm approaching rapidly, Joseph drove me to Grant Hospital on his way to a meeting of Chicago Pediatric Society of which he was President. He did not want me to be stranded at home in a blizzard.

The admitting clerk put me in a clean Surgical Ward because the Obstetrical Ward was full. Joseph objected to this, but there was no other space available. He made us promise, however, if I did go into labor, they would move me immediately to a labor room. But I was having no pains so Joseph went on to the meeting.

Dr. Falls was called and he ordered the usual method for inducing labor, at that time, quinine until my ears rang, followed by four ounces of castor oil. I was in the bathroom when the nurse brought the large glass of oily liquid.

I tried valiantly to swallow it, urged on by the encouraging nurse. I immediately vomited and the bag of waters broke all over the bathroom floor. A new way to induce labor! And it really started with a jolt — severe cramps every three minutes.

They trundled me over to the elevator and into a labor room

immediately. None too soon, for the pains kept increasing at more frequent intervals.

I kept glancing at the clock on the wall, timing my pains. They were nothing compared to the agony of my first delivery. In fact, I was enjoying the normal progression of the baby going down the birth canal. Dr. Falls arrived just in time to deliver the baby's head and to do an episiotomy under local anesthesia. He congratulated me on having a nine pound, three ounce baby through a justo-minor pelvis.

"Of course, the second baby is usually easier," he pointed out.

I wondered why he had warned me so sternly not to have a second child, but I guessed he was overprotective, since he was such a good friend of my parents. Anyhow, I was supremely happy that the pregnancy and labor had turned out so well.

After I was returned to my room, my first thought was to call Joseph. It was then midnight, but I didn't think he was asleep because the Chicago Pediatric Society meetings usually lasted until after eleven.

He picked up the phone after two rings, "Hello," he said quietly.

"You have a nine pound, three ounce baby girl!" I blurted out.

"What?" He was amazed. "That's impossible. You could not have had a baby without me!"

I laughed. That remark was so typical of his scientific skepticism.

"Well *impossible* or not I did it! I did not want *you* to go through labor pains again."

There was a long silence. The new father was speechless. Then he said, "You are something else Dorothy. Get some sleep. Goodnight dear."

As I snuggled into the hospital pillow I thought, "That's the only time he ever called me *dear*." It was worth it.

Ellen was pure gold. She never looked or acted like a

newborn. At over nine pounds she seemed almost a month old and usually ate and slept on her own schedule as contented as a kitten.

Joanne liked her from the start and since Mrs. Carlson and I had made her feel as an auxiliary little mother, she soon leaned to hold Ellen's bottle and take her for little strolls in the back yard.

As Ellen grew up, Joanne's group of girl friends made a living doll out of her. One of their favorite games was *dress and undress Ellen*, who just loved all the attention — but sometimes it got out bounds. One day, I unexpectedly returned from my office early to find the whole group of seven year-olds playing hospital with Ellen as the patient.

"What are you all doing?" I said. Then I saw an enema bag being held up in the air by Dede while Joanne was trying to insert the tip of the rubber hose into Ellen's vagina!

Joanne, in a play nurse's uniform answered innocently, "Oh we're just giving her an enema. She needs it! Her bowels haven't moved for a week!"

I picked up Ellen whose face by then was beet red from her efforts not to be *a cry baby.*

"But they'll never play with me again!" she wailed while I carried her off to the safety of my bedroom.

The sad part of it was that there were no little girls Ellen's age on the block, only three little boys and Joanne's tribe of Lois, Dede, Myra, Ruth and Margaret. So Ellen became a tag-a-long, that is, until she discovered that the three boys were fun.

She bossed them constantly and they loved it. She received three engagement rings; a rubber washer from the butcher's son, a plain dime store ring from the boy down the block and an elegant jeweled peacock, little finger ring swiped from his mother's jewelry case by Michael, the son of a shoe salesman.

I thanked Michael for his pretty present but naturally insisted that he give it back to his mother. She substituted a less expensive engagement ring.

When I asked Ellen how she could be engaged to three four year olds simultaneously, she answered, "Oh it's easy. Each one thinks he's the only one."

And so began a love career in spite of my attempts at educating her about faithlessness.

The children gave me wonderful new outlets for my creative nature. I often tied this in with my medical career, as when I decided to hold a benefit performance of children's dance.

I built a little theater in the basement with an outside entrance, exit and footlights. It had rows of folding chairs and I obtained a City Permit to hold public performances there.

I choreographed my own Mid-Summer Night's Dream to Mendelssohn's music and spent many happy hours training my children and their friends in primitive ballet steps. Their mothers made the costumes.

The two high points of the performance were Joanne's solo on her toes; and Ellen and Michael's pas de deux.

When the performance was over, the cast presented me with an orchid. I was thrilled, but somewhat deflated when Michael's father announced in a loud voice, "I hope I never see my son in pink tights again!"

When Joseph was asked how he liked giving a benefit performance for the Chicago Heart Association in his basement he replied, "It would have been more financially remunerative for the Heart Association if we had given them the money outright." As usual, I had not figured out how much building a little theater would cost!

The income from the sale of tickets at one dollar a piece had been fifty dollars and the labor and materials for constructing the theater over two hundred dollars. Poor Joseph, he would never become rich with a wife like me.

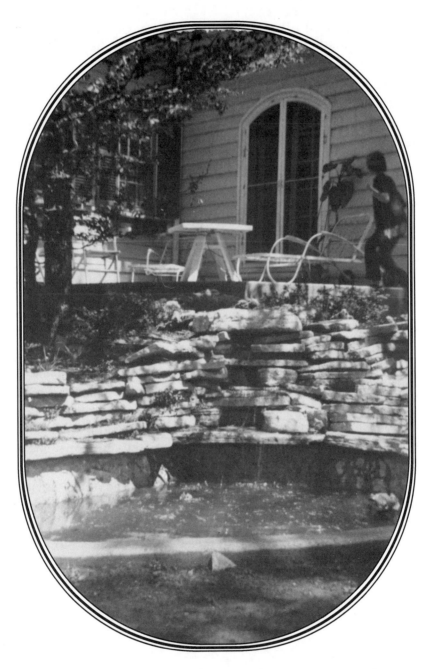

Goldfish pond surround by quarry rocks

GYPSIES, GANGSTERS AND GUNS

I could scarcely believe so many years had passed since I was worried about starting pre-med courses at Urbana. I never thought then, that someday, I would be the teacher.

I'd been teaching at the Stritch School of Medicine, Loyola University, Chicago, since 1936, but it was my second teaching appointment in 1948, that pleased my father the most; Associate Clinical Professor of Pediatrics at the University of Illinois, College of Medicine. This entailed teaching junior medical students in groups of five or six for an entire day once a week. I thought it would be practical to expose them to a day in a pediatrician's life.

We met at Grant Hospital for rounds in the Premature Station and on my private and charity patients. Then, after lunch in the hospital cafeteria, we spent the afternoon at my office. Most of the boys — I did not have any young women students the first year — were very attentive and seemed to enjoy this experience. However, one of them could not have cared less about learning. He spent all his time looking out of the windows.

I became annoyed by his rudeness. If he was bored, at least he could have pretended not to be. I decided to call on him.

"Now, doctor," I asked, "here is a new mother who has a baby with a severe diaper burn. How do you suppose she is washing his diapers?"

"I have no idea," he shrugged off the question immediately.

"What would you tell a mother about getting the right pH in the diapers?"

"I have no idea," he repeated.

"Let's pretend you are in your office and a mother presents such a problem. How would you know what to advise her? You obviously have not been listening to my instructions to this mother."

"I would not need to know," he answered glibly.

"Why not?" I asked.

"Because all I'd have to do is walk into the next room and consult my Dr. Spock," he said smugly.

This nettled me so I said, "Well since Dr. Spock has all the answers, why don't you go home and read him right now." He left sheepishly and received a D for the Pediatric Outpatient hours.

After office hours, the remaining five medical students squeezed into my Buick convertible and made house calls with me. On the way to the last call, one of them asked plaintively, "Are all your days like this? I'm bushed!"

I laughed, "Oh, this was one of the easier days."

They all groaned. Then one said, "I don't think I want to be a pediatrician. I read somewhere it's the second most hard working and poorest paid specialty of all."

"Well, you'll never get rich being a pediatrician but think how many young lives you'll improve. Besides it's such fun."

They still looked doubtful and I often wondered how many students I had inadvertently dissuaded from becoming baby doctors by our spending a typical day in a pediatrician's life. I really enjoyed teaching these young people. Although I was fifteen years older than most of them, it made me feel young again to be with them and hear their naive remarks.

About that same time, a second important appointment was offered to me. The Medical Director of Grant Hospital asked if I would take the position of Director of Medical Education. I accepted and became the first DME Grant ever had.

The duties of this office were to arrange all medical programs for the edification of the medical staff. The most important function was sorting out of the applicants for internships and residencies.

Men and women who did not qualify for positions in the large hospitals applied to smaller ones, such as Grant. There were many foreign students who applied and, by trial and error, I found that certain medical schools produced better trained individuals. I made up lists of these medical schools rating them on a scale of one to ten. This helped in getting a smooth running intern-resident program.

Since I was responsible for the interns' actions, I felt as though I were a combination of mother confessor and Dean of men and women. One especially bright intern, Mariano Tan of Chinese ancestry, was more like a son to me than any of the others. Joseph and I invited him each Thanksgiving and Christmas to have dinner with us and the girls and the whole family took him to our hearts. We called him our "adopted son" and he never abused the privilege.

When he married a pretty little Filipino nurse he asked me to be his "mother " at the Catholic ceremony. Again I had to take that long walk alone to the altar ahead of Bella and her foster father.

We gave the newlyweds and their guests a Chinese brunch in Chinatown and pictures from that became one of my cherished possessions, especially the one of Mariano catching Bella's garter and looking very embarrassed.

Besides these new appointments, I was still Attending Pediatrician at Grant, as well as Director of the Premature Station, plus continuing in my private practice. In those days, doctors still made house calls and most nights would find me, after having put in a full days work, trying to locate a patient's home.

It had been a particularly busy day at my office, with patients bawling and their inquisitive mothers asking long list of questions, mostly about non-essential details. So, even though I was on my way to make three house calls, it was a pleasant relief to be cruising along the Outer Drive between the ruffled Lake and the smooth lagoon.

I turned off the drive, away from the tall apartment buildings fronting the Lake, onto a commercial through street with taverns on three corners out of four.

My street guide informed me that Frontier Street was 635 West. It was narrower than an alley and after passing it once, I had to make a U turn to come back to it. It was a blind street, the sign warned at the entrance, but I drove into it anyhow parking in the shadow of the elevated structure. This was in the depths of a slum worse than any I had ever visited before.

There were no names on the doors, no numbers and no bells, so I knocked on the nearest door with more determination than I felt. It opened under my hand and I was faced with an extremely dirty, narrow and winding uncarpeted staircase. It seemed almost completely vertical. I climbed up slowly, hoping I would not slip or drop my doctor's bag. I tried knocking at the only door at the top of the stairs. It opened a crack and was shut immediately. I knocked again. This time a voice questioned my identity.

I was annoyed by now and answered brusquely, so the door was opened in haste. I passed through a kitchen crowded with people and entered a dingy living room.

Carefully I placed my coat on a metal chair, having learned from my clerkship in OB that there are hidden inhabitants in overstuffed furniture.

One of the dark-skinned women called out to someone in the bedroom and she entered carrying a baby that appeared to be about two weeks old. She looked extremely worried. The grandfather explained she had lost a newborn a year ago from choking on its feeding.

The mother was in her late teens with the luscious beauty of a ripe peach. As she took her breast out of her unbuttoned dress and inserted the nipple in the baby's mouth, I felt a strange incongruity between her primitive appearance and the artificiality of her surrounding. She should have been sitting under a palm tree at the edge of a jungle, natural, wild and free.

Mucus was running from the infant's nose but his temperature was normal and his throat was not infected. All other findings including his breath sounds were normal.

My diagnosis was *anxious mother*.

I spent fifteen minutes or so reassuring the young mother, refused the dollar offered in payment of the house call and went out, carefully navigating down the steep, dirty stairs. Imagine living like that, with ten or more people crowded into three rooms.

The next house call was on Gregory Godla, a five week-old infant who I had great difficulty locating, there being no numbers on any houses in his block. The first door I knocked on was opened wide and immediately an iron-faced man of about fifty asked me to come in without answering my questions as to whether the Godlas lived there. Apparently they didn't for the apartment was bare of furniture and there was a sinister stillness about the empty rooms with most of the light shut out by brown wrapping paper pasted on the windows.

The man said nothing, merely stood and looked at me. I hastily left. He followed me in his shirt sleeves, into the dampness of the street and called, "I find the Godlas for you. Come!"

I felt much safer following behind him, down some stairs into a basement below a basement. The man had disappeared and in his place staring with the same insolent eyes was a large gray alley cat. I knocked at the door he was guarding and after a few minutes a disheveled man with mussed hair and no shirt, stuck his head out of the door.

I told him who I wanted to see.

"A baby?" He gave a great hoot of laughter. "There ain't no kids in here. Ain't that right, Baby?" he said over his shoulder to someone inside.

She came to the door; a caricature of Sadie Thompson. She had long bleached blonde hair hanging over her shoulders and had her hands on her hips. I caught a glimpse of an upright cream colored piano outlined against a bright rose wall.

"What are you, a nurse?" Her shrewd, but sad, eyes scrutinized my hat, coat and bag. "A doctor?" She was more friendly. "Maybe you'll find that baby in the Cuban village two doors north."

I found a door over a tavern where a juke box going full blast. I knocked as loudly as I could for inside there were many sounds: an electric guitar, some boisterous singing, a shrill female arguing and several children crying fortissimo. I knocked several times more, still there was no answer. I climbed another rickety flight of stairs.

A laconic man in dirty underwear directed me with one hairy thumb to another door. I pushed the door open, went down a dim hall and entered a kitchen where there were eight women, five children and six freshly killed chickens.

A man stumbled sleepily out from the bedroom. Where there had been bedlam there was now silence. I was being appraised, even by the children. Then, the sick baby was pushed out in his dirty satin basinett. The rest of the children who huddled around him were brushed away like flies and the examination began.

The mother seemed concerned, but not unduly so. As I discovered signs of illness in the baby, a red throat and fine râles in the chest, she would translate my findings into Spanish to the enlightenment of the audience. She was definitely enjoying her role in the performance and punctuated her remarks with long exhaled puffs of cigarette smoke.

When I informed her that the baby would need a penicillin shot, she fled sobbing into the bedroom and all the women followed her. The lone man remained, pale and shaken.

No one would hold the baby. Finally one little ten year-old girl volunteered. She said she liked seeing people get shots. She held the baby in a strong grip and received a lollipop as reward. Immediately, the other children were back clambering for lollipops also.

The third house was even more dilapidated than the other two. From the outside with no glass in the windows and with one or two boards across the staring eye sockets of the empty window frames, it appeared more like a rookery for winter crows than a human habitation.

The stairway had no rail, strewn garbage covered corners of each landing and there were no doors on any of the apartments. The cold wind blew violently against the boards over the open windows.

Three stories up I found my patient, a two year old boy. His mother was frightened. His father was young and angry. They had some difficulty at the free Clinic and had been asked to leave. They were gypsies, most unwelcome in any clinic because of their reputation of picking up anything handy.

The baby had been crying for days with an ear ache and the cold wind did not help. What good was medical care in this situation?

I had to push the hovering parents away. They seemed to be trying to protect the baby from my examination.

"You will have to let me look at him!" I said sternly. "I cannot tell what is wrong with him unless I do."

"OK," said the father drawing his wife away, "but no shots."

By this time I was thoroughly exasperated. "What kind of a Specialty am I in?" I thought. First, I have trouble finding these rat traps and then, I have to fight families for the privilege of looking at their dirty children.

I examined the struggling two year old. I dreaded examining this age group most of all, because they were strong and too young to reason with. It was the "no" age. He had tonsillitis and ear infection.

The father picked up the prescription I had written and accompanied me down the excuse for stairs. I managed the top flight by not looking down. I had always had a great fear of heights and with nothing to hold on to I felt unsteady.

The gypsy took my arm.

"Do not be afraid. I won't let you fall."

All at once my resentment against the unfortunate soul faded away.

When we reached the street I said, "How far is it to the drugstore?"

"About five blocks."

"Get in my car and I'll drive you there, unless you have a car."

The young man sighed hopelessly and shrugged.

"Who has a car these days?" he asked.

"Just a moment." I said. "I might have some samples." I felt in the side pocket of my doctor bag. Fortunately I had an antibiotic and a bottle of ear drops.

I explained the directions I had written on the prescriptions to the father. He offered to pay me for the visit now that he did not have to buy the prescriptions. I just shook my head.

How could I charge these poor people? I thought of a conversation I'd had with my neighbor, Mrs. Gershey, a believer and promoter of Communist propaganda. She'd chastised me for being materialistic and promised, "I'll have your big house for my Headquarters one day, and you and your husband will have to give free health care to the poor."

I smiled as I drove home to the house that was supposed to be the Communist Headquarters for her block.

The next evening, my one house call was located in a well-to-do neighborhood where most of my patients lived.

At least I won't have to worry about being helped down any rickety stairways, I thought. Little did I know that what was in store would prove even more harrowing.

It was dark in the vestibule of the apartment building and, just as I was peering at the names beneath the door bells, I had an eerie feeling that someone was standing behind me.

I looked over my shoulder and saw two men close by. I instinctively knew they were going to rob me. Suddenly I had a brilliant idea.

"I'm trying to see on which floor the Silversteins live," I said helplessly. "They have a very sick child and I cannot see which bell to ring. I am their doctor."

I guess I caught them off guard. It was enough to make them pause for some time and finally, after looking at one another, the larger man shrugged his shoulders and got out the flashlight. He found that Mrs. Silverstein lived on the third floor. They rang her doorbell.

I thanked them profusely and was quite relieved to hear the lock on the security entrance to the stairs released. What I did not like was that the two men followed me up to the third floor. Fortunately, Mrs. Silverstein had the door open. I threw myself through it and quickly slammed it shut.

Mrs. Silverstein's eyes were big question marks.

"Did those men follow you in?" she asked.

"I'll bet they don't live in this building, do they?"

"I've never seen them in my life," she confirmed.

I told her the whole story. I was shaking.

After examining and treating my patient, I was a bit hesitant about leaving. I said, "I hate to be a coward, but I really did not like the looks of those men. Their expressions reminded me of some of my gangster patients. Their eyes were so dead looking."

Mrs. Silverstein said she did not like their looks either.

"If you'll wait a little while until Steve gets home, he will escort you to your car."

I was relieved and while I was waiting, I told Mrs. Silverstein about several experiences I had with the underworld.

One day, I made a house call in an Italian neighborhood. I knocked and knocked on the front door of a nice looking brick house. The door opened a crack and a small middle-aged man with a large barking German Shepherd stood, peering out anxiously. He opened the door when he saw who it was, but had difficulty restraining the fierce animal, who looked as though he would dearly love to take a bite out of my neck.

I asked the father to put the dog in another room while I examined the child. I had battled protective dogs before who had taken a dim view of my approach to their little charges. All went well with the visit except for the end of it, when I told the parents that the child would have to be hospitalized for possible rheumatic fever. Naturally, they were greatly disturbed but I was not prepared for the father's belligerent attitude.

"You'll take good care of her won't you, Doctor?" he said.

"Oh course." I answered.

"I don't mean ordinary care. I want the best! Don't spare the cost."

By this time I was getting a little annoyed.

"I treat all my patients the same way regardless of cost. They all get the best that medicine can offer!"

That *dead look* appeared in the man's eyes.

"You make her well, do you hear me? Or it will be very bad for you. Do you understand?"

I said I did and left quickly before I lost my temper. I was glad I had not told the man to get lost, because, just one week later, I saw the headlines, GANGSTER AND DOG KILLED.

The article said that the machine gun killing had taken place in the same doorway of the brick house I had visited.

Chicago, at that time, was the site of many ruthless assassinations. But this was not the only place the gangsters had invaded. My own beloved Northwoods was the setting for another story I shared with Mrs. Silverstein.

I had been on vacation from my internship when my father awakened me around midnight.

"Get your bag, Dorothy, we are going to make a house call."

"Why? Where?" I was still half asleep and quite bewildered.

"Don't ask so many questions. Get dressed right now! Hurry up!"

I automatically obeyed him as usual but my heart gave a little jump when I saw a .32 revolver sticking out of his belt.

We got in the old Buick and followed a sleek sports car onto County Trunk I and then branched off onto a grass covered, private road near a small lake.

The car we were following disappeared. We got out of our car in front of a ramshackle log and frame structure. I hesitated. Father, who had gone up to the open door, turned and said, "Come on. What are you waiting for? Bring your bag with you."

We passed through a series of rooms without any halls. It was very quiet in these empty rooms. The only furniture was a few tables, chairs and some cots.

In the last room of all, a pale man with a terrified expression was lying on his side with his thighs drawn up over his abdomen. He was moaning softly and rhythmically.

I counted his pulse, took his temperature and blood pressure and gently felt his abdomen. He winced with pain. His abdomen had *board-like rigidity* a medical term describing a condition resulting from free blood in the peritoneum.

He was acutely tender over his spleen.

I asked him, "Did you fall on your belly?"

He nodded, "I fell off the running board of a car."

"How long have you been like this?"

"Three days, ever since another doc gave me a shot for pain."

"Did it help?"

"Just for a few hours."

"Well, you are in serious condition and have to go to the hospital at once! Do you have a phone here?" Foolish question − a phone in a hide out?

"When your friends come back have them get an ambulance and take you to a hospital in Superior or Duluth right away. I think you have a ruptured spleen!"

"Can't I wait for my mother to get here?"   She'll be here tomorrow morning."

"Of course not, every hour cuts down on your chances. Your pulse is week, your temperature high and your blood pressure is low."

The man kept arguing. I answered, "Man, you're in shock! If you want to wait until your mother arrives, she will find a corpse."

This finally pulled him up short. At last, he was convinced. I gave him a shot of morphine and we left.

On the way back home my father drove slowly, puffing on his pipe and thinking. I wondered why he was so quiet. Finally I said, "A penny for your thoughts, Father."

He glanced at me quizzically, raising one eyebrow. I had never seen him look at me quite like that.

"My thoughts are worth more than a penny to you I imagine."

"Why?"

"Because I've suddenly realized who you really are. You have grown up into a real physician. That took guts back there."

It was a long time before I got back to sleep. That was the greatest compliment my father had ever given me.

The following summer, while I had been recuperating from my illness, a man who looked familiar appeared on the verandah of the Lone Larch cottage.

"Don't you know me, Doc?" he said. "You saved my life?"

I asked him to sit down. He looked strong and healthy. I thought, "The devil must have protected him."

"That sure was a close call." he said. "The doctors weren't sure I'd make it until they pumped ten pints of blood into me and took out my spleen. They told me that another two hours would have been too late. My mother came up to the hospital the next day and never left my bedside for a week."

"Well, I'm glad to know what happened to you."

"But that's not what I came for. I want to pay you." And he pulled out a thick roll of bills.

I shook my head, "You don't owe me anything."

The man insisted, "I want to pay you. Don't you think my life is worth something?"

I did not answer that question because, if I had been truthful, I would have answered, "No!" Instead I said, "I cannot accept a fee since I don't have a Wisconsin license."

This convinced him, but he still wanted to repay me in the only way he could. He handed me a slip of paper with a telephone number on it.

"Well, here's where you can reach me day or night. If ever I can do you a favor, just let me know." And after shaking hands, he left.

I joked with Mrs. Silverstein, "So you better treat me nice or I'll sic my gangster friend on you."

Just then Steve arrived and escorted me to my car. He waited until I drove off.

I wish that gangster had been around when those two men followed me upstairs.

PALM SPRINGS

Many years had gone by with the girls graduating from college, getting married and Ellen having two boys. Joanne had three step-children and a thriving Physical Therapy practice.

I missed the girls who were living far away, so I threw myself into hard work with disastrous results. I had recurrent pneumonia and the last bout did not clear up for six weeks.

As I looked out of my bedroom window at the leaden skies and the dirty snow, I longed for the warm sunshine and lovely flowers of Palm Springs. "If only I felt stronger, I'd go out to Desert Manor where we used to spend Christmas vacations when the girls were going to high school and college, I dreamed. Then the thought of the long walk through the airport discouraged me. Why I could barely make it to the bathroom without getting exhausted!

I discussed it with Joseph. He could see how discouraged I was so he said, "My head resident of a few years ago has a practice in California. He is visiting his parents here and planning on returning to Los Angeles soon. You remember him, Manny Schneider?"

I indeed remembered him, a charming, bright pediatrician with a most intelligent wife. I called him up at his parents' home. He came over and encouraged me to make the trip. He would obtain a wheel chair at the airport. "You won't have to walk a step," he said. "You'll never get well in this foul Chicago weather."

I felt better already with the prospect of Palm Springs appearing like a mirage in front of me.

I asked Joseph anxiously whether he could manage without me. "What do you mean, professionally or domestically?" he asked, smiling.

"How about both?"

"I surely can manage both practices, if that's what you mean now that we have a good assistant. About the home part of it," he chuckled, "you aren't much good in your present condition anyhow!"

I threw a sofa pillow at him. "You know how to hurt a girl," I laughed.

So it was all set. I extended my leave of absence from Grant's Baby Clinics, my position as Director of Education and my teaching position at the University of Illinois.

Kay, the faithful nurse from our office, came over and helped me pack. She had tears in her eyes as she said, "I have a terrible feeling that once you get out in California, you won't want to come back. What will we do without you at the office?"

I smiled, "Oh, you'll manage with the charming Dr. Goodman.

Kay shrugged her shoulders. In her slightly biased opinion there were only two superlative pediatricians in the world, Dr. Joseph Greengard and Dr. Dorothy Welker.

"I'll be back," I said. "I cannot desert Dr. Joseph."

Kay looked sad and unconvinced as she finished packing two large suitcases and my carry-on bag. "Why do you want so many clothes if you're coming back right away?" She really was suspicious.

"Well, I do want to be completely well when I return or this darn infection will recur. I've had it twice before you know."

Kay had to admit that was true and gave me a long good-bye hug.

The trip went well. Manny could not have been more

considerate and when we reached the Los Angeles Airport, he turned me over to Father Vincent, my daughter Ellen's uncle by marriage. He was a slender white-haired priest who had performed Ellen and Jack's wedding ceremony.

He had a dilapidated old Dodge with a heater stuck in the "on" position. I thought I would die as I lay in the back seat for the three hours it took to get to Desert Manor. My temperature was up and, with the warm dress I wore, I was sure it had reached at least 104 degrees.

But as soon as Father Vincent turned me over to Mrs. Sullivan, the owner of the resort, I relaxed. Mrs. Sullivan reminded me of Nanny. Heavy set, bossy and efficient, she helped me undress, take a shower and get into bed. She even unpacked my dresses for me.

I fell asleep and awakened twelve hours later feeling much better. However, there was one drawback to the Desert Manor. The cottages were in a circle surrounding a large patio with windows and porches opening out into a small separate garden. Sound carried easily in the clear air. Even a soft sneeze in one of the units could be heard in all the rest. Any argument had an immediate appreciative audience.

I was bothered by a nagging cough, very loud and frequent, which was much worse at night. No sooner would I lie down than it would start — cough, cough, cough long into the night. That did not bother me, except that I worried I would keep the neighbors awake. And the more I coughed, the more I worried. The more I worried, the more I coughed . . . a vicious cycle.

Finally after a week of this torture, I called a real estate agent who Mrs. Sullivan had recommended.

She was a chic, attractive red head of about my age and we liked each other immediately. Her name was Geri Thompson, a divorcee' with a delightful sense of humor.

I explained my problem and asked Geri if she could find me a rental house where I could cough to my heart's content without anyone hearing me.

She told me she had just the place and we drove three blocks away to a charming house with three bedrooms, two baths, a large living room with a dining area, a good sized kitchen and breakfast nook overlooking a huge pool, with the mountains for a backdrop. And best of all, it had a wood burning fireplace.

I said, "I'll rent it!"

Geri laughed, "You cannot take the first thing I show you! I'm not earning my money that way. By-the-way, it's six hundred a month plus utilities, but it has an option for buying. Let's go look some more."

"I don't want to see any more, I love this place. How much does the owner want for it?"

Geri said, "$37,500 unfurnished, $42,500 furnished."

I called Joseph as soon as she left.

"Oh Joseph, I've found just the house for us. You must fly out and see it. You'll love it!"

A long silence, then Joseph's sensible voice saying, "Dorothy, you've fallen in love with houses all over the United States and Europe. What are we supposed to do with this one when we don't have our California licenses?"

"I know it sounds crazy, but you have to see it to appreciate it. Please come out and look at it. Besides I'm lonely." I knew that would persuade him, if nothing else did.

Joseph sighed. He knew he was being manipulated, but he could not resist the invitation. He was rather lonely too.

"All right", he said. "I'll let you know when I can get away."

I told Geri I wanted her to meet him. We had lunch at one of her favorite restaurants to celebrate and she helped me move into the new house the next day.

I was delighted with the new home. It was completely furnished even to the pretty dishes and Mexican pottery calendar with a Sun God on it. I could hardly wait for Joseph to see it. Would he turn it down the way he had done so many other houses?

He arrived the following weekend looking tired and

"citified." I greeted him warmly, but he had a wariness about him that he always had when he knew I wanted something. Once he'd said to me, "You have everyone fooled except me." It was a joking remark.

When we drove into the circular driveway with our rented car, I saw his expression lighten.

He likes the front yard, at least. Wait until he sees the inside of the house and the pool, I thought.

It was a happy house, built by a contractor, for himself, with 3 x 6 studs instead of 2 x 4's and everything in cedar. The interior color scheme was orange, yellow and sage green throughout and it lifted Joseph's mood when he walked in.

I showed him through the place being careful not to talk because I knew how my superlatives always turned him off. But I could not restrain myself when we opened the sliding-glass kitchen doors.

"And here is the best of all, the back yard with an eight foot concrete block wall and a 40 x 24 foot pool. We'll also have five citrus trees — all bearing!"

"Oh, we will, will we?" he teased.

I was afraid I had gone too far.

"What do you think?"

He liked it but did not want to raise my hopes too high so he said grudgingly, "It's very nice but would you want to buy it now?"

My heart beat faster with my suppressed, "Yes, oh yes!" but I knew I had to make some semblance of being sensible so I said, "Well, I thought we could rent to the down payment of buying it if we liked it."

Joseph nodded his head. He never said much so when he nodded a "yes" it was like another man effusing for fifteen minutes.

I gave him a big hug and then cooked the first meal for him in the workable kitchen. It turned out a lot better than the first one I had cooked thirty years ago. After all, I had quite a lot of practice since then.

So a week later, we moved into our new home. I was in seventh heaven.

The California State Board for licensing physicians was notoriously difficult. It had to be that way because so many doctors wanted to practice there. Many of my friends had taken it numerous times and failed. A lot depended on the attitude of the examinee. If one appeared cocky and talked down to the examiners, it meant an immediate failure. After all, since it was an oral examination, they did what they wanted.

I was terrified of any examination and this was no exception. I had studied three months for it and, when the day came, I was shaking. Joseph and I were walking over from our hotel to the L.A. County Building where the exam was being held.

"Aren't you scared?" I asked. I knew that was a stupid question because I had never seen him frightened in all the years of our married life.

"What of?" he parried, knowing full well what I meant.

"Of those creatures in there just waiting to eat us?"

He laughed, "You make them sound like monsters."

"They are! They are just trying to get rid of all competition. That's why they flunk so many."

"Don't worry, Dorothy. If we were intending to practice in Los Angeles or its suburbs, we would have less of a chance. There are too many pediatricians and general practitioners now. In Palm Springs, there is only one pediatrician and although the population has a predominance of retired persons, there are eight thousand children, mostly offspring of working people. They need us."

I felt a little more comfortable, but later, waiting to be called in seemed endless. I went in before Joseph. He squeezed my hand for good luck.

I was ushered into a huge empty room with five men seated

behind a bare table. I sat down opposite them placing my hands, palms down, on the table in front of me. I could feel the perspiration cause my hands to stick to the varnish. The examiners were polite, cordial even. They asked me why I wanted to practice in Palm Springs. I told them about my recurrent attacks of interstitial pneumonia and the last one that had refused to clear up.

They asked numerous questions that had nothing to do with pediatrics. I hoped I answered them correctly. Then one doctor, with very sympathetic eyes, said, "Now tell us all about interstitial pneumonia."

I could have kissed him for he knew that, since I had suffered with the disease, I must have studied up on the history, the etiology, physical signs, laboratory findings, treatment and prognosis which I described in that order.

When I was through all five men nodded their heads simultaneously and excused me. Just before I left I asked, "When will I get the results?"

The Chairman of the Examining Board smiled and quietly said, "In about three months, but I wouldn't worry about the outcome if I were you."

I thanked them all gratefully and left. I had stopped shaking.

Joseph was inside for such a long time that I wondered about it. When he came out, he was grinning broadly.

"What happened?" I wanted to know when we had left the building.

"They asked me such involved questions that it took a long time to answer them and when I finished, one of the doctors said he had learned more pediatrics in that half-hour than he had learned in all of medical school."

I could well believe it, since I remembered all of Joseph's medical writing besides the many brilliant lectures he had given. I was so proud of him.

So we bought the house before we received the official notice that we had passed the California License Examinations and we were never sorry we did. We practiced there, happily, for twenty-five years.

~ 1974 ~

Joseph had to be at County Children's Hospital for another year-and-a-half, while I commuted back and forth between Chicago and Palm Springs.

Every night in Palm Springs, before I fell asleep, I would take an imaginary trip turning off County Trunk I outside of Minong, Wisconsin, onto the one quarter mile, narrow road lined with jack pines. Then, I would take a sharp turn near the lake and suddenly there it was, my own clearing. To the right, I saw the breathtaking beauty of a hundred tall Norways standing ankle deep in fragrant needles just where my father had planted them forty years ago. To the left were the log covered ice house, garage and wood shed straight in a row blending their weathered paint into the foliage of the hill behind them. These visions were my lullabies, soothing me to sleep.

In the summer, I took Ellen and the two grandchildren to my beloved Lone Larch Cottage. Now instead of daydreams the beautiful vision was reality with the family driving down the lane to the Lone Larch cottage.

We were a mixed bag of three generations, my daughter, her two sons ages eight and ten and I. We all were excited. To me this was superb and before I unpacked my bags I had to run to the top of the stairway leading sixty feet down the steep embankment to the lake. I inhaled the fresh water scents which came up in a welcoming cloud to fill my desert-starved senses.

The boys could not get into their cut-offs fast enough for a plunge into the spring fed lake, but I was satisfied just to sit at the top of the stairs and breath in the mingled odors of balsam, wintergreen and wild roses, taste a blueberry or two and run my hand over some reindeer moss growing beside the banister.

Our Wisconsin home was located on the shore of a three mile long lake shaped like a pipe, the house being sixty feet above the water level on the bowl. The nearest cabin that I could see was a mile across an unbroken expanse of clear water. In the center, the deepest depth equipment had never touched bottom, leading to a local myth that Lake Gilmore was the site of an extinct volcano. More likely, Lake Gilmore, like most of the lakes in the region, had been gouged out by an advancing glacier in the ice age.

Whatever the cause, it made a cool home for large walleye and northern pike until it was over-fished. Now the challenge of fishing was even greater because a catch was such a rarity that a fish of any decent size was a real prize.

Our rods, reels and tackle boxes, all carefully hidden in the attic had to wait until more important things were done. Things like unpacking, making supper and connecting the TV. In my mind, there was nothing more important than getting fishing tackle ready for use at a moment's notice.

I told Merril, our handyman, not to put up the signs with my name on since I wanted to have a few days to enjoy myself. Originally, I had not practiced in Wisconsin in the summer, but when I obtained my Wisconsin license and the news spread, people began to find their way to my back door.

The nearest doctor was twenty-six miles away, so it was not so flattering that more and more summer residents sought me out. Finally, in desperation, since they were coming at all odd times, I put up a sign reading, OFFICE HOURS 2 - 4 PM EXCEPT SUNDAYS.

I regretted this later, because it curtailed my fishing time. It concentrated the flow of patients to the afternoons, but, of course, did not account for accidents or high fevers in children.

But I felt sorry for those campers and resorters who became panicky when their children became ill or hurt themselves so far away from their favorite doctor. I revamped the forty-by-twenty foot rumpus room in the basement to make a reception and examining room. It turned out well with its Honduras mahogany paneling and a native stone fireplace all across one end of the room. Merril had hauled the stones for it from the bottoms of all the rivers he had fished. For years he had been noting each uniquely colored, shaped and textured rock. When the time came to build fireplaces, he volunteered to gather them up.

A funny, but almost tragic, thing happened concerning his good deed of rock gathering. There had been a few break-in's and enterings around the lake so the Greengards had made a convenient arrangement with our neighbor, the Wilsons, whose road we shared. We promised that after we left and they heard someone drive into our common road, they would call Paul Berg. Paul would pick up his shotgun and drive over in his Bronco.

The plan worked very well. The Wilsons heard a truck drive in. They called Paul, who arrived posthaste to our lodge clearing. In the pitch dark he heard some peculiar knocking noises. Fortunately he, being a cautious soul, called out "Who's there?" If he had not, Merril would have had his pants full of buck shot as he innocently unloaded the last truckload of fireplace rocks.

Merril never drove in our driveway again without first notifying the Wilsons.

I was very tired after the long trip from California. Merril carried my bags to the upstairs bedroom. Since the house was perched high on the hill overlooking the lake, my room had a floating quality. In addition there were three sets of double casement windows which opened inward in the most intriguing way.

Growing tall next to the windows were two twenty-foot jack pines, one to the North and one to the East. As I lay supine on the four-poster bed, I could almost touch the branches of the trees. I could join in the intimate life of a family of chipmunks and spy on chickadees, rose-breasted grossbeaks and yellow goldfinches as they hopped, unconcerned, from branch to branch. They preened their feathers and scratched their ears, completely oblivious to the fact that I was peering at them from the other side of the screen. Of course one quick movement of mine and they were gone.

If I were perfectly still, though, I could observe them for an hour at a time, which I did, much to the detriment of a carefully drawn up schedule I had vowed to follow. Every year, I made the same good resolutions and, every year, I ended up with a broken schedule.

The chipmunks were more wary than were the birds. They tilted their heads and glanced over their shoulders as they clung to the rough bark. Their bright eyes were ever-watchful that my little Austrialian silky dog, Centa, would not see them. They ran down the tree at the slightest sound.

The north bedroom was fairly large, but still it was dwarfed by my grandmother's dowry bed which occupied two thirds of it. This hundred and fifty year-old four-poster was made of honey colored pear wood with pawn shaped posts. They had rough tops where the canopy, not long gone, had once perched.

When Grandma Welker came as a bride from her family's farm to Grandpa's house in Red Hill, Pennsylvania, she brought with her the usual dowry; her bed, linens and a dresser to store them in. The dresser, a Pennsylvania Dutch, lovely, hand-carved piece of fruitwood, was inlaid with darker walnut and paneled with one half-inch line of black at the edges of the inlay.

In the old days, there were no springs, just ropes stretched between knobs on the bed frames. The old beds were short, because most people were short, so my father had lengthened the bed with six inch pole-wood inserts in the frame and cut the legs off an equal amount. Even so, the bed still had to be climbed into and there was room for a trundle bed underneath. I imagined my tiny grandmother must have needed a ladder to get into her bed.

It was a complete mystery to me how such a diminutive, barely five-foot tall, woman could have raised four children, spun, wove, knitted and sewed all their clothes, kept a vegetable garden by herself, made soap, helped with the slaughtering, pickled, canned, dried all kinds of produce and had time to help out in the General Store attached to the thirteen room house in Redhill.

Of course, she did not play bridge, go to cocktail parties, travel, play golf or serve on committees, as I and so many of my friends did.

But, as I lay on the four poster, I thought of how much this bed had meant to Grandmother − being part of her dowry and where all her children had been conceived and delivered. Both she and Grandfather had died in this bed and all at once I felt the fourth dimension of time closing in on me. The timeless trees and the timeless bed posts wrapped their arms around me and rocked me to sleep.

The brown and black-striped chipmunk ran up the north tree as Centa spied him from her perch at the end of the bed. She barked violently and the day began.

Well, hopefully, I can unpack and straighten up the house a bit before the patients arrive.

I was mistaken. Just as I was putting the first tempting bite of poached, country fresh egg in my mouth, I heard the rapid, loud knocking on the front door. I knew it was urgent by the rapidity of the knocks. A couple of well spaced sounds almost always meant something not too serious, but a staccato stream of knocks signified an actual crisis, at least one in the mind and emotions of the knocking patient.

This was a fish hook emergency. Outside the screen door stood a husky father, with a two day growth of beard, holding a towel over the hand of a frightened eight year old.

I steered them to the basement and office door — thinking regretfully of the unpacked boxes littering the place. No time to get settled before the stream of injured started. "The Welker Emergency Room," as Joseph called it — was open for business, whether it was ready or not.

The little fellow was speechless, bug eyed and shaking, his freckles standing out distinctly over his pale cheeks.

I gasped when I removed the towel. I had never seen such a big hook in such a little hand.

His father said, "Sure, him and his brother must have been fishing for whales! I've never seen that hook before."

It was about two and a half inches in size with at least one half inch buried in the fleshy base of the boy's thumb. As usual it was an on-the-pier injury. In all my experience with fish hooks, I had only about ten percent of them occur in boats. Many of them happened when two or more children were casting off a pier, probably because they were standing close together. And for some reason it seemed to happen to brothers.

"Another dangerous place for getting tangled up with the wrong end of a bait," I told the father as I cleaned off Bobbie's thumb, "is in a sporting goods store. When an absent minded customer looks away as he is reaching for a bait hanging on a rack, there's a good chance the first thing that a plug catches will be a human being."

"Will it hurt?" Bobbie asked.

Since I never lied to patients, I told Bobbie the truth. I showed him the bottle of procaine and as I drew up the medicine into the syringe I explained the *Welker Method*, which I had invented. I put the needle into the opening by the hook and followed along the course of the metal, injecting as the needle went deeper. "This is the only pain you will feel," I told him.

He nodded his head and held his hand out trustfully.

I thought, There is nothing more appealing than a believing child. I always prayed I wouldn't betray that trust.

As I waited for the local anesthetic to work I wrote his

history on one of the 3x5 note cards I kept my mini-records on in the Country Office.

Name: Bobbie Sullivan
Father: James
Local Address : Jenkins Resort, Lake Gilmore, WI.
Home: Aurora, Illinois
Age: 8-years-old
Birthday: June 9, Normal Delivery
No serious illnesses or operations
Last tetanus shot: 3 months previous

I was glad of that – I wouldn't have to stick him twice.

His father spoke up. "He's a brave boy!" he said with obvious pride.

I asked, "Are you all nice and numb, honey? Can you feel this?"

His father sat beside him on the examining table and steadied Bobbie's arm against his own. Bobbie said he could not feel a thing as I grasped the end of the hook and guided it along the anesthetized channel. It came along fairly easily because, fortunately, the barb was not too large. The difficult part of the maneuver was at the curve of the hook but after a bit of strenuous tugging, out it came barb and all.

I much preferred this to the old method of pushing the hook through the skin and cutting off the barb, as that produced two holes and besides (heaven forbid!) it ruined the hook often attached to a favorite lure.

Bobbie was smiling as I placed the hook on his good palm.

"Save this for whales," I said and felt than his smile was worth more than any fee his father could have paid me.

When the patient left, I finished my breakfast, wondering if there was anything worse than a cold poached egg. I then hurried back down to the basement to unpack.

I liked to pack if I were going someplace where I wanted to go, but unpacking was a real pain. There never was enough room in which to put all the contents of the boxes. Why in heaven's name had I sent all this junk? Would I ever be able to use it all? Or had I just been trying to get rid of all these samples which were flooding my Palm Springs Office?

Well, anyhow, here they were and I dreaded arranging them on the edge of the book shelves already two-thirds filled with medical and non-medical books. All at once, I thought of my elder grandson, Joel. At the moment, this ten year-old was intrigued by my office which was ordinarily "off-limits" to him and his brother. He was a gifted child and eager to learn.

I thought that, like Tom Sawyer, maybe I could make my work appealing enough for him to want to volunteer. But I had to make him think I was not suggesting it, so I went upstairs.

Ellen had made a ruling which once and for all solved the problem of "What shall we do now, Mama?" The edict was that mornings were made for work and afternoons for play. In this way playtime was at a premium and too precious to be wasted in contrast with the morning drudgery of pulling up weeds in the garden. I added a little bribery with the payment of a quarter for each day's work well done, beds made before noon, clothing picked up and gardening done without too much prodding on the part of the adults.

Joel, as usual, was procrastinating as to starting the gardening chores. He was lounging at the breakfast table, making faces at his milk. When I appeared, he straightened up.

"What was wrong with the patient?" he wanted to know.

"Oh, just the biggest fish hook I ever saw, I said casually.

"Gee, how neat? Did you keep it?"

"No, but if you finish your milk I'll show you one almost as big!"

Never had milk disappeared so rapidly. He was bounding down the stairs to the basement, followed by barking Centa who hoped another patient was arriving.

The fish hook was oohed and aahed over with the moral plainly visible about piers and brothers when suddenly I said, "Well, here are all these medicines to be sorted."

The fish rose to the bait.

"How do you do that?"

"I put the cough medicines on one shelf, the antibiotics on another and the eye drops, ear drops and nose sprays on another."

"Can I do that?" He never wanted to help, but rather just wanted to do the job himself. I was reluctant.

"How could you sort them?"

"Oh, I'd put all the same labels together and if I don't know what something is, I'll ask you." His face was illuminated with desire to do something just a little beyond him, a new experience, a challenge!

"OK, but be sure the rows are straight and that you don't break anything."

About an hour later, we heard footsteps on the inside stairs. Joshua, Joel's eight year-old brother, wandered into the office in his usual carefree way.

"What are you doing here?" asked Joel wrathfully. "You're supposed to be weeding!"

A hated chore, most definitely.

Josh opened his eyes innocently: "Oh, I just came down for some insect repellent. The gnats are awful. What are you doing here?"

"I am arranging Nonnie's samples."

Looking at me, Josh said, "Gee, I wish I could help."

Here was a predicament — two helpers when I needed only one. Also I did not want Joel's newly acquired importance to be destroyed. I looked at him. He was steadfastly examining the samples, sorting medicines industriously.

"Do you think there is anything Josh could do right now?" I asked him.

"W-e-l-l," said Joel doubtfully.

There was a long silence while Josh sat down waiting for the verdict. It was hard to have a big brother who always decided everything.

"W-e-l-l, maybe you could carry the empty boxes out to the wood shed."

Josh was delighted. He had escaped weeding. All that morning his little legs trotted up and down the stairs, out to the wood shed and back.

By lunch-time, with a little sweeping and dusting by Ellen, the reception and examining room looked habitable. Best of all, the samples were arranged in shining, sorted rows by a happy young man who had decided to be a doctor.

All was set for a pleasant summer at Lone Larch cottage, yet I could not sleep for the longest time that night. For some reason my whole life was unrolling before me. Almost like drowning, I thought.

From my girlhood in Pennsylvania through my four pre-medic and four medical school years, on through my internships, my illness, my lovely three months in the Northwoods, residency, my work at the World's Fair, my happy courtship and marriage, my three offices and two darling daughters and my grandchildren – my entire life to that point had been so full and exciting.

Even the battles of a woman doctor fighting prejudices against *hen medics* seemed worthwhile.

As I finally felt myself drifting off to sleep I wondered, What will happen next?

Could the rest of my life's journey possibly be as stimulating and productive as it had been so far?

Only time would tell.

THE END

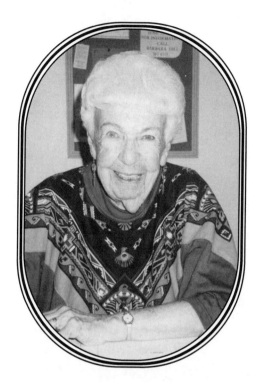

Dr. Dorothy Welker is still going strong at age 91. She resides in Arizona and Wisconsin, and continues to renew her license to practice medicine in Wisconsin, though she no longer sees patients. "It keeps my mind sharp," she says.

No doubt writing her second book is keeping her on her toes as well. If you would like to know when Dr. Dorothy's next book is available, send us a postcard with your name, address and telephone number and we'll put you on our mailing list (we do not provide/sell our lists to anyone else). We'll also be happy to forward any letters to Dorothy.

Judith James, President
Paper Moon, Inc.